Workbook for

PRACTICAL MICROBIOLOGY

Workbook for
PRACTICAL MICROBIOLOGY

SECOND EDITION

Upasana Bhumbla
MBBS MD (Microbiology)
Infection Control Officer and Assistant Professor
Department of Microbiology
Geetanjali Medical College and Hospital
Udaipur, Rajasthan, India

Forewords

TV Rao
FS Mehta

JAYPEE
JAYPEE BROTHERS MEDICAL PUBLISHERS
The Health Sciences Publisher
New Delhi | London | Panama

Jaypee Brothers Medical Publishers (P) Ltd

Headquarters
Jaypee Brothers Medical Publishers (P) Ltd
4838/24, Ansari Road, Daryaganj
New Delhi 110 002, India
Phone: +91-11-43574357
Fax: +91-11-43574314
Email: jaypee@jaypeebrothers.com

Overseas Offices

J.P. Medical Ltd
83 Victoria Street, London
SW1H 0HW (UK)
Phone: +44 20 3170 8910
Fax: +44 (0)20 3008 6180
Email: info@jpmedpub.com

Jaypee-Highlights Medical Publishers Inc
City of Knowledge, Bld. 235, 2nd Floor
Clayton, Panama City, Panama
Phone: +1 507-301-0496
Fax: +1 507-301-0499
Email: cservice@jphmedical.com

Jaypee Brothers Medical Publishers (P) Ltd
Bhotahity, Kathmandu, Nepal
Phone: +977-9741283608
Email: kathmandu@jaypeebrothers.com

Website: www.jaypeebrothers.com
Website: www.jaypeedigital.com

Workbook for Practical Microbiology

First Edition: 2018

Second Edition: **2019,** Reprint: 2024

ISBN 978-93-5270-562-7

Printed at

Dedicated to

My Guruji

Grandparents

Parents and my beloved Sisters

whose blessings and encouragement have always
been with me throughout my endeavor

Foreword

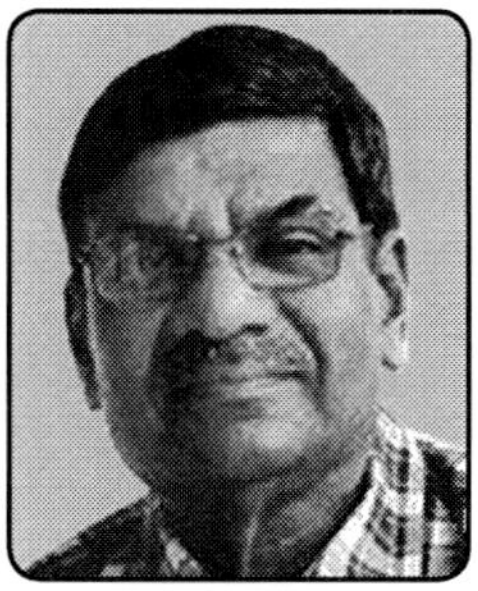

I am happy and delighted to write the Foreword for the second edition of *Workbook for Practical Microbiology* by Dr Upasana Bhumbla, Infection Control Officer and Assistant Professor at Geetanjali Medical College and Hospital, Udaipur, Rajasthan, India. In this edition, she has included didactic ideas for practical microbiology to be practiced by both undergraduates and postgraduates. It also adds up to the idea of bringing one book associated with many innovative chapters for learning. Chapters ranging from General Microbiology which addresses the basic concept in microbiology, to newer concept of Applied Microbiology are very well written in this workbook. The content of the book is to make our best efforts to train the medical graduates and how to lead a better understanding of the complex topics, thus to improve the quality of diagnostic microbiology.

I congratulate her for this comprehensive work and wishes for great success and her continuous efforts to bring forth such a book for students.

TV Rao MBBS MD (Microbiology)
Professor of Microbiology
Travancore Medical College
Kollam, Kerala, India
Faculty of e-learning at Infection Control Academy of India
Hyderabad, Telangana, India

Foreword

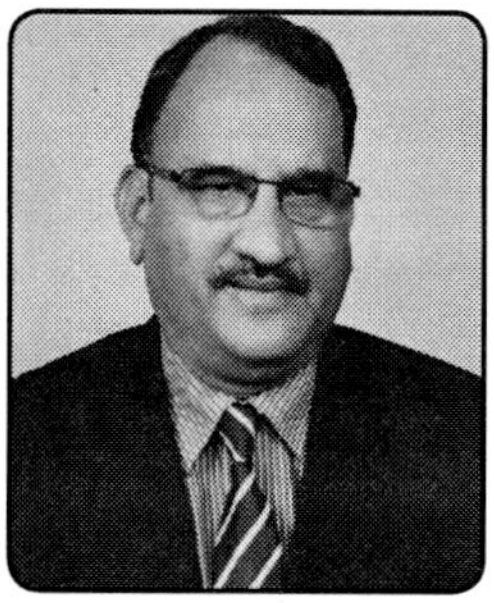

I am happy to know that the second edition of *Workbook for Practical Microbiology* is released. First edition was widely appreciated among faculty and students all over India. This book is fully updated with a simple lucid presentation style. I acknowledge this practical manual compiled by **Dr Upasana Bhumbla**, Infection Control Officer and Assistant Professor, Department of Microbiology, Geetanjali Medical College and Hospital, Udaipur, Rajasthan, India, under the guidance of **Dr AS Dalal**, Professor and Head, Department of Microbiology at Geetanjali Medical College and Hospital.

The book is ideally recommended for medical students and junior doctors who are preparing themselves for various examinations.

FS Mehta MBBS MS (Surgery) FIAS
Dean
Geetanjali Medical College and Hospital
Udaipur, Rajasthan, India

Preface

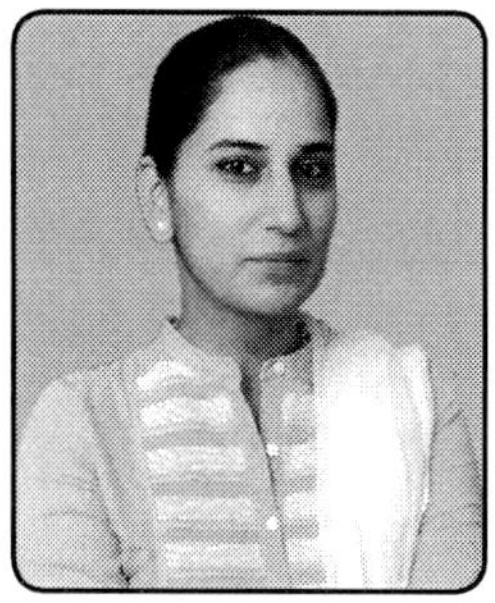

The intent of the book *Workbook for Practical Microbiology* is to provide a workbook for the practical exercises in microbiology which covers all the important topics. This book has been designed in a pattern to help students, learn and work on the practical and clinical aspects of microbiology.

I, therefore, undertook this endeavor based on my experience of teaching undergraduates. For the benefit of students, the likely questions and short notes that are important in the practice of medicine have been included. This book teaches the concept in a workbook style so that the students are able to understand and write the practical notes. The recent advances that are increasingly applied in the rapid diagnosis of infectious diseases have also been included.

Upasana Bhumbla

Acknowledgments

I acknowledge the following persons for reviewing this manual:

Anuradha Sharma
Associate Professor, Department of Microbiology
All India Institute of Medical Sciences
Jodhpur, Rajasthan, India

AS Dalal
Professor and Head, Department of Microbiology
Geetanjali Medical College and Hospital
Udaipur, Rajasthan, India

Balramji Omar
Additional Professor, Department of Microbiology
All India Institute of Medical Sciences
Rishikesh, Uttarakhand, India

Dinesh Raj Mathur
Dean and Professor, Department of Microbiology
Shadan Institute of Medical Sciences
Hyderabad, Telangana, India

FS Mehta
Dean and Professor, Department of Surgery
Geetanjali Medical College and Hospital
Udaipur, Rajasthan, India

Gyaneshwari
Professor, Department of Microbiology
Shadan Institute of Medical Sciences
Hyderabad, Telangana, India

Sarbjeet Sharma
Professor and Head, Department of Microbiology
SGRD Medical College and Hospital
Amritsar, Punjab, India

Shobha Paul
Professor and Head, Department of Microbiology
MNR Institute of Medical Sciences
Hyderabad, Telangana, India

I am thankful to Shri Jitendar P Vij (Group Chairman), Mr Ankit Vij (Managing Director), Mr MS Mani (Group President), Ms Pooja Bhandari (Production Head), Ms Samina Khan (Executive Assistant to Director-Content Strategy), and their team especially Mr Samir Khan, Ms Seema Dogra, Mr Jagvir Singh and Mr Narsingh Kumar of M/s Jaypee Brothers Medical Publishers (P) Ltd, New Delhi, India, for helping me in compiling this book.

I am also thankful for the following sources and references that helped me a lot while revising the contents of book:

1. www. wikimedia. org for figures for Chapter 1.
2. www. healthessentials4you.com for Chapter 2.
3. Forber BA, Sahm DF. Weissfield diagnostic microbiology. Bailey and Scott's Diagnostic Microbiology, 13th edn. Missouri, Mosby Elsevier. 1998:238-42. For Chapter 11.
4. Washington CW, Stephen DA, William M, et al. Koneman's Colour Atlas and Textbook of Microbiology, 6th edn. Philadelphia; Lippincott's Williams and Walkins. 2006:68-74. For Chapters 11 and 12.
5. Miles RS, Amyes SGB. Laboratory control of antimicrobial therapy. In: Gerald Colle J, Barrie P, Andrew GF, Anthony S (Eds). Mackie and McCartney Practical Medical Microbiology, 14th edn. New Delhi. 2007:151-78. For Chapters 12 and 14.
6. Parija SC. Textbook of Microbiology and Immunology, 3rd edn. New Delhi; Elseiver RELX India Pvt. LTD. 2016: 102-6. For Chapters 2 and 15.

Department of Microbiology
Geetanjali Medical College and Hospital
Udaipur

PASSPORT SIZE
PHOTO

NAME : --

FATHER'S NAME: --

DATE OF BIRTH: --

PERMANENT ADDRESS: --

TELEPHONE: --

EMAIL ID: --

REGISTRATION NUMBER: --

DATE OF JOINING: --

SIGNATURE AND SEAL

HEAD OF DEPARTMENT

Student Index

Head

Department of Microbiology

Chapter 1 History of Microbiology

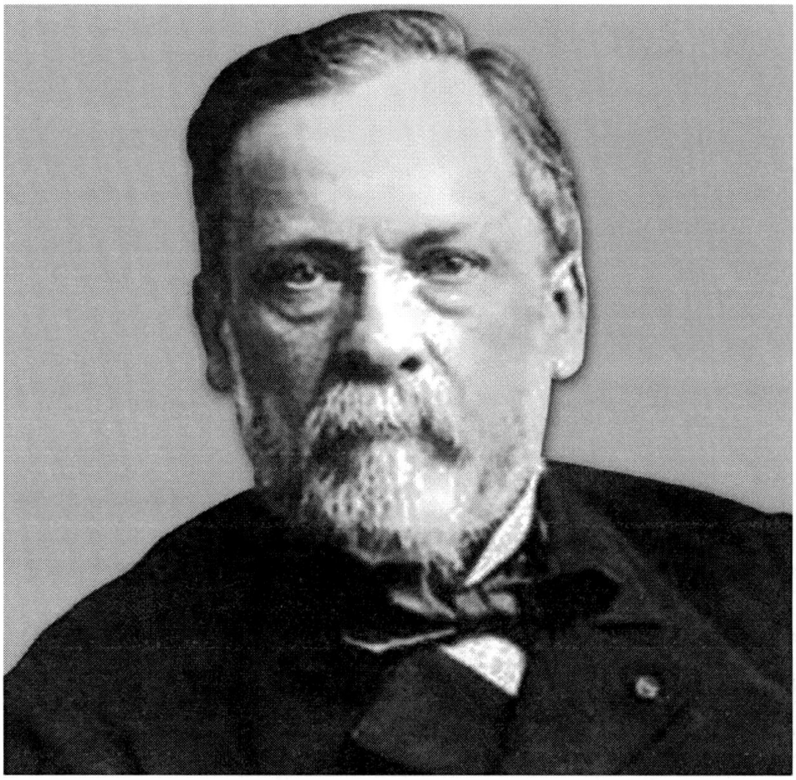

Louis Pasteur (Father of Microbiology)

IMPORTANT CONTRIBUTIONS

Louis Pastuer known as 'Father of Microbiology' (1822-1895)

- He was a professor of chemistry in France. His studies on fermentation led him to take interest to work in Microbiology
- He had proposed the principles of fermentation for preservation of food.
- Introduced sterilization techniques and developed steam sterilizer, hot air oven and autoclave
- Described method of pasteurisation of milk
- Contributed for vaccine development against several diseases such as Anthrax, Cholera and Rabies
- Postulated "Germ theory of disease".
- Introduced liquid media concept
- Founder of Pasteur Institute, Paris

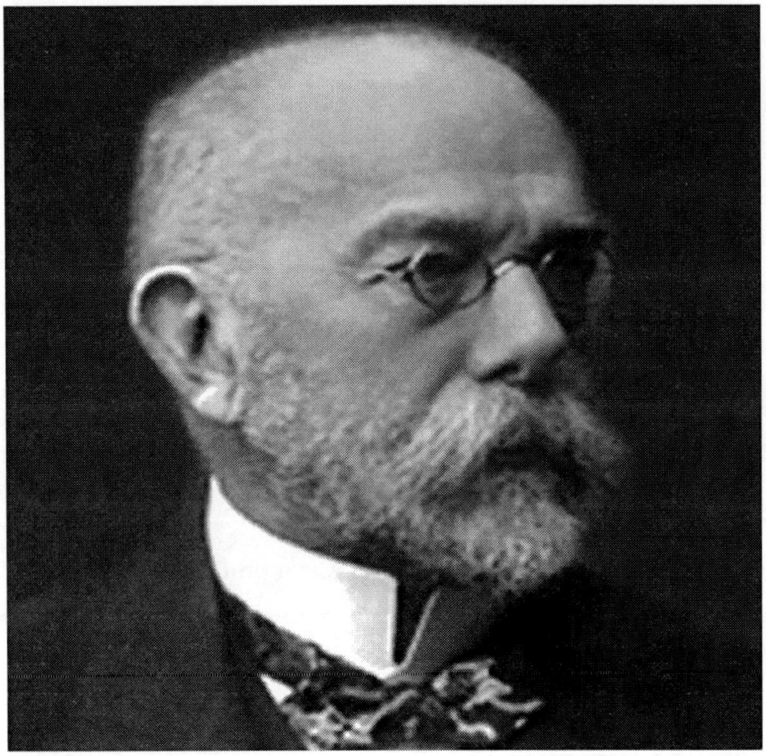

Robert Koch (Father of Bacteriology)

IMPORTANT CONTRIBUTIONS

Robert Koch known as 'Father of Bacteriology' (1843-1901).

- He got Nobel prize in year 1905 for the discovery of tubercle bacilli
- Introduced solid media for culture of bacteria and use of agar
- Methods of isolation of bacteria in pure culture
- Described hanging drop method for motility of organism.
- Discovered bacteria like Anthrax, Cholera and Tubercle bacilli
- Introduced staining techniques by using aniline dyes
- Koch's postulates and Koch's phenomenon was given by him

KOCH'S POSTULATES

1. The microorganism should be constantly associated with the lesion.
2. It should be possible to isolate the organism in pure culture from the lesion of the disease.
3. The same disease must result when the isolated microorganism is inoculated into suitable laboratory animal.
4. It should be possible to re-isolate the organism in pure culture from the lesions produced in the experimental animals.
5. Antibody to the causative organism should be demonstrable in patient's serum

Exceptions of Koch's postulates: Some bacteria that donot satisfy Koch's postulates are ***Mycobacterium leprae*** and ***Treponema pallidum***

KOCH'S PHENOMENON

Robert Koch observed that guinea pigs already infected with tubercle bacillus developed a delayed hypersensitivity reaction when injected with tubercle bacilli or its protein.

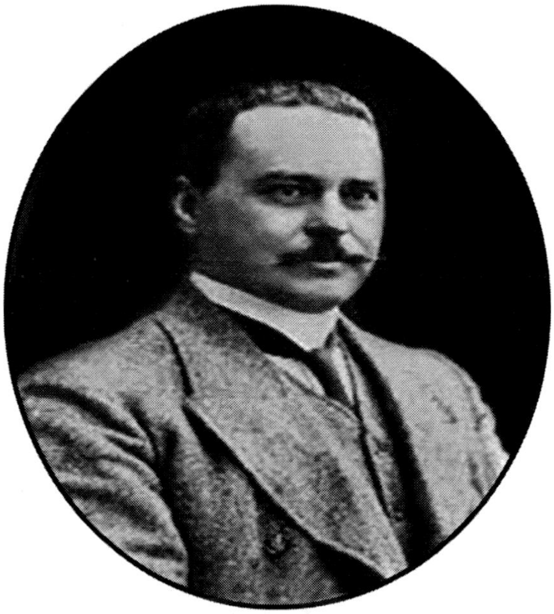

Sir Ronald Ross

IMPORTANT CONTRIBUTIONS

Awarded Noble prize in the year 1902 for his contribution for development of life cycle of malarial parasite in mosquito

- Ross developed mathematical models for the study of malaria epidemiology
- Established the developmental stages of malaria parasites in anopheline mosquitoes; and described the complete life cycles of *P. falciparum, P. vivax* and *P. malariae*

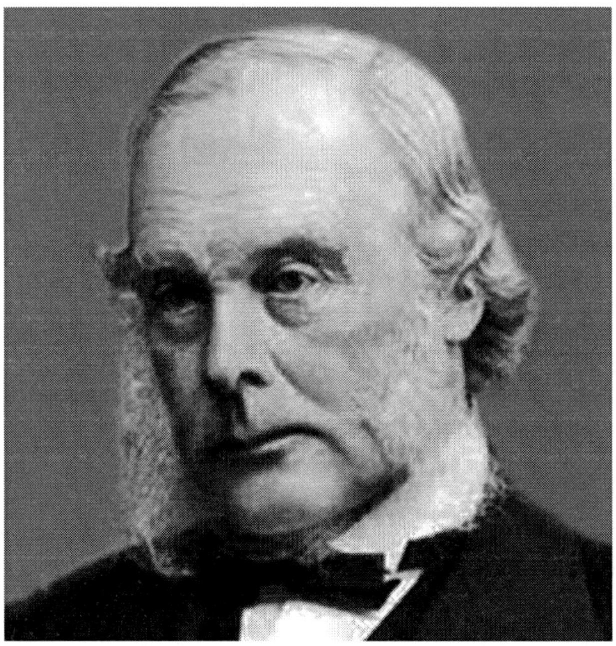

Joseph Lister

IMPORTANT CONTRIBUTIONS

Joseph Lister known as 'Father of antiseptic surgery'

- Observed that postoperative infections were greatly reduced by using disinfectants such as diluted carbolic acid during surgery to sterilize the instruments and to clean the wounds.
- He instructed surgeons under his responsibility to wear clean gloves and wash their hands before and after operations with 5% carbolic acid solutions.

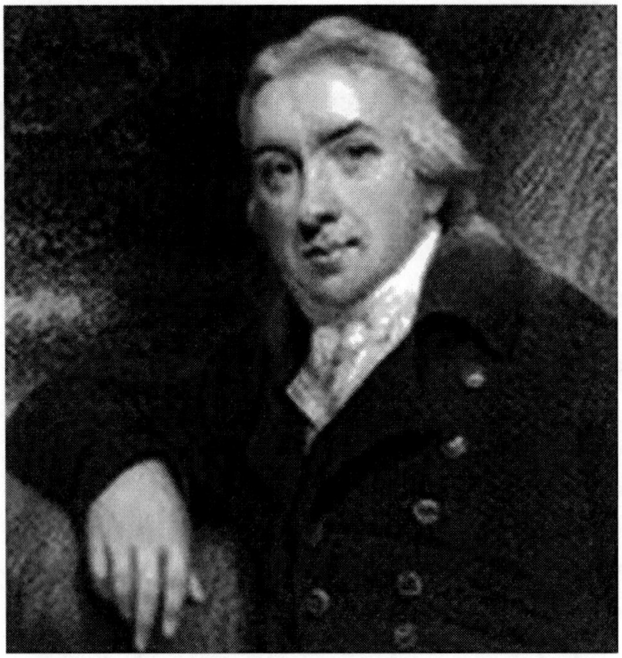

Edward Jenner (Father of Immunology)

IMPORTANT CONTRIBUTIONS

Edward Jenner known as 'Father of Immunology'.

- Developed the first vaccine of world, the small pox vaccine.
- Used cowpox virus (Variolae vaccinae) to immunize children against smallpox from which the term 'vaccine' was derived

NAME FEW NOBEL LAUREATES

1.

2.

3.

4.

5.

Chapter 2 Microscopy

A COMPOUND MICROSCOPE IS PROVIDED WITH DIAGRAM AND LABELLED PARTS

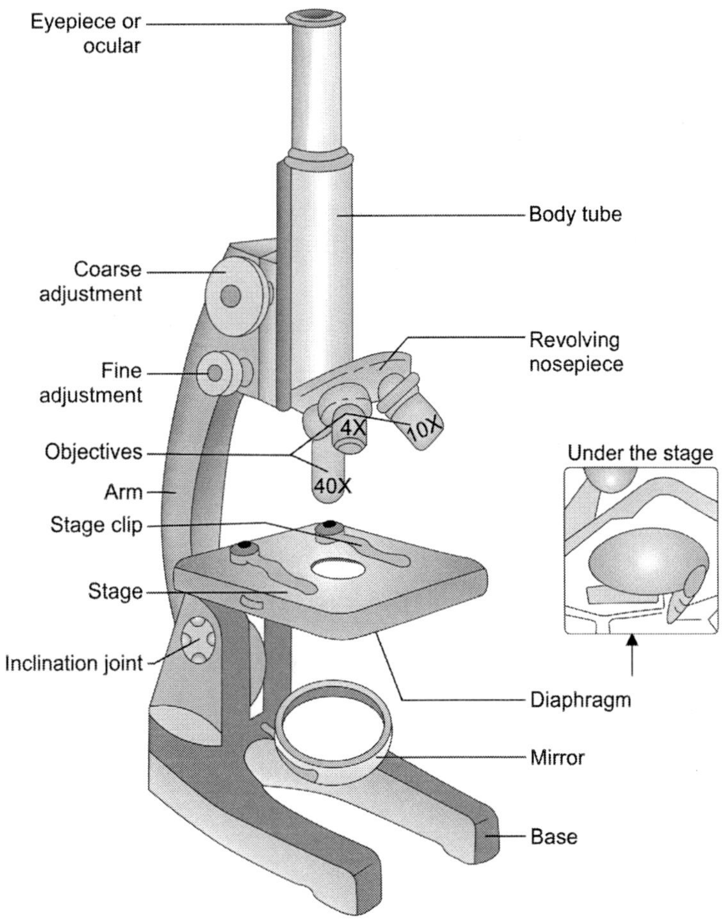

Q1. Enumerate the various types of Microscopy. Add a note on the principles involved.

A. Light Microscope

Principle:

The rays emitted from light source pass through the iris diaphragm and fall on the specimen. Light rays passing through the specimen are gathered by the objective and a magnified image is formed.

B. Dark Ground Microscope

Principle:

Object appears bright against a dark background, which is done by use of dark field condenser. Dark field condenser has a central opaque area that blocks light from entering the objective lens directly and has a peripheral annular hollow area which allows the light to pass through and focus on the specimen obliquely. Only the light which is reflected by the specimen enters the objective lens whereas the unreflected light does not enter the objective. As a result specimen is brightly illuminated, but the background appears dark

C. Phase Contrast Microscope

Principle:

Condenser has a central opaque area with a thin transparent ring, which produces a hollow cone of light. Some light rays are bent due to variations in density and refractive index within the specimen. Undeviated rays strike a phase ring in the phase plate, while deviated rays miss the ring and pass through rest of the plate. The phase ring is constructed in such a way that the undeviated light passing through it is advanced by one-fourth of wavelength, deviated and undeviated waves will be about half wavelength out of the phase and will canel each other when they come together to form an image

Light rays go through → condenser → specimen → phase ring → objective lens → ocular lens

D. Electron Microscope

Discovered by Ernst Ruska in 1931. An electron microscope (EM) uses accelerated electrons as a source of illumination.

Principle:

The electron beam is focussed by circular electromagnets, which are analogous to the lenses of light microscope. The object is held in the path of beam scatters the electrons and produces an image which is focussed on a screen. As the wavelength of electrons used is approx. 0.005 nm, the resolving power of electron microscope is 100,000 times than that of light microscope (0.1 nm)

Two types are:

Transmission electron microscope
Scanning electron microscope

Specimen preparation: Specimen to be viewed under EM should be able to maintain its structure when it is bombarded with electrons. Steps required are

Fixation: Cells are fixed by using glutaraldehyde or osmium tetroxide for stabilisation

Dehydration: Specimen is then dehydrated with organic solvents

Embedding: Specimen embedded in plastic polymer, hardened to form a solid block.

Slicing: Specimen cut in slices by an ultachrotome knife, which is mounted with copper.

E. Fluorescent Microscope

Principle:

Fluorescent dyes are exposed to UV rays, they become excited and are said to fluoresce i.e. they convert the invisible, short wavelength rays into longer wavelength (visible light). The fluorochromes emit light of a given wavelength when excited by incident light of a different (shorter) wavelength. To view this fluorescence in the microscope, several light filtering components are needed.

Specific filters are used to isolate the excitation and emission wavelengths of a fluorochrome. A dichroic beam splitter (partial mirror) reflects shorter wavelengths of light and allows longer wavelengths to pass. A dichoric beam splitter is required because the objective acts as both a condenser lens (excitation light) and objective lens (emission light); therefore the beam splitter isolates the emitted light from the excitation wavelength.

This epi-illumination type of light path is required to create a dark background so that the fluorescence can be easily seen. The wavelength at which a beam splitter allows the longer wavelengths to pass must be set between the excitation and emission wavelengths of any given fluorochrome so that excitation light is reflected and emission light is allowed to pass through it. A bright light source producing the correct wavelengths for excitation is also required for fluorescence microscopy, normally a mercury arc lamp.

Q2. What is a simple microscope?

Q3. What is a compound microscope?

Q4. What factors constitute the magnification of a compound microscope?

a. **Total magnification in low power**

b. **Total magnification in high power**

c. **Total magnification in oil immersion**

Q5. What is the Resolving power and numerical aperture of a microscope

a. **Resolving Power :**

b. **Numerical aperture :**

Q6. How will you focus the given compound microscope?

a. **To visualize a hanging drop preparation/Wet preparation of stool:**

b. **To visualize stained smears:**

Chapter 3 Sterilization and Disinfection

Q1. What is the thermal death point of a microorganism?

It is defined as the temperature at which all organisms of a culture will be killed by heat either instantaneously or within an arbitrary brief finite period.

Q2. Define

a. **Sterilization:** It is a process by which all living and dead microorganisms, including viable spores are either destroyed or removed from an article, body surface or medium.

b. **Disinfection:** It refers to the process that destroys or removes all the pathogenic organisms.

c. **Antiseptic:** It is an agent that can be safely applied on the skin or mucous membrane to prevent infection by inhibiting the growth of bacteria.

Q3. Enlist the factors influencing the efficacy of disinfection

Q4. Classify the different methods of sterilization.

A. Physical methods:

1. **Sunlight**
2. **Heat**
   a. **Dry heat:**
   Red heat, flaming, incineration, hot air oven

   b. **Moist heat:**
   At temp below 100°C—Pasteurization, Inspissation, Vaccine Bath

   At temp 100°C—Boiling, Tyndallization, Steam sterilizer

   At temp above 100°C—Autoclave
3. **Ozone**
4. **Filtration**
5. **Radiation**

B. Chemical methods:

- Alcohols
- Aldehydes
- Phenols
- Halogens
- Oxidising agents
- Salts
- Surface active agents
- Dyes
- Gases

Q5. Mention the method of sterilization for each of the following:

1. **Test Tube:** Hot air oven
2. **Cystoscopes and endoscopes:** 2% Glutaraldehyde
3. **Surgical dressings and linen:** Autoclave
4. **Disposable catheters and disposable gloves:** Gamma radiation
5. **Rubber gloves:** Autoclave
6. **Disposable syringes:** Gamma radiation, 10% ETO
7. **Glass syringes:** Hot air oven
8. **Pipettes:** Hot air oven
9. **Clinical thermometers:** Isopropyl alcohol
10. **Basal media and Sabouraud's Dextrose Agar:** Autoclave
11. **Loeffler's serum slope:** Inspissation
12. **Lowenstein Jensen's medium:** Inspissation
13. **Sugar media:** Filtration
14. **Inoculation loop:** Red heat flaming
15. **Forceps and scalpel:** Hot air oven and flaming
16. **Scissors and needles:** Hot air oven, flaming

17. **Serum and other body fluids:** Vaccine bath

18. **Antibiotic solutions:** Filteration and ionizing radiation

19. **Vaccines:** Vaccine bath

20. **Dental equipment:** Autoclave and ethylene oxide (ETO)

21. **Suture material:** Autoclave and Ethylene oxide (ETO)

22. **Plastic endotracheal tubes:** 2% Glutaraldehyde, Gamma radiation

23. **Heart lung machine:** Ethylene oxide, 5% cresol

24. **Soiled dressing:** Incineration

Q6. How are the following places sterilized and methods involved?

1. **Operation theater:**

2. **Sick rooms and wards:**

3. **Virus laboratories:**

Q7. What is

1. **Inspissation**

2. **Intermittent sterilization or tyndallization**

Q8. What are surface active agents.

Q9. What are gaseous agents.

Q10. Define pasteurisation. Describe the different methods.

Chapter **4**

Laboratory Instruments

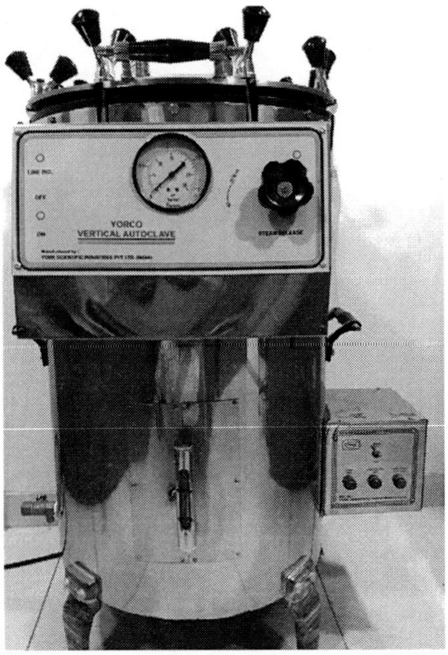

1. Autoclave

Principle:
Water boils when its vapour pressure equals that of surrounding atmosphere. When atmospheric pressure is raised, boiling temp. is also raised.

Sterlisation conditions:
121°C for 15 mins at pressure of 15 pounds (lbs) per square inch (psi).

Uses: For surgical instruments, culture media, autoclavable plastic containers, Plastic tubes and pipette tips, solutions, biohazardous waste

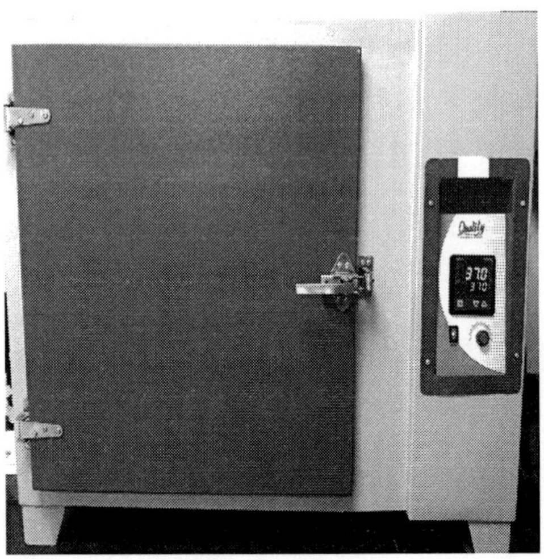

2. Incubator

In biology, an incubator is a device used to grow and maintain microbiological cultures or cell cultures.

The incubator maintains optimal temperature, humidity and other conditions.

For routine bacterial cultures, temperature is mainted at 37°C.

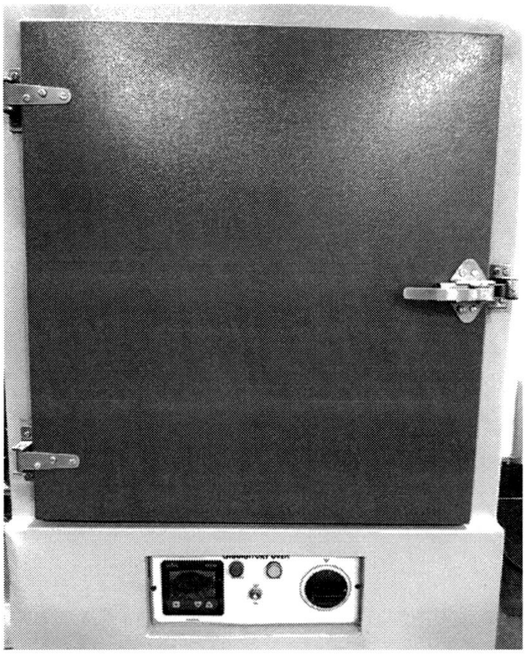

3. Hot air oven

Widely used method of sterilisation by dry heat.

Temperature:
Holding temp. of 160°C for 2 hours is requied for sterilisation

Materials sterilised:
Glassware like glass syringes, petri dishes, flasks, pipettes and test tubes

Surgical instruments like scalpels, forceps

Chemicals life paraffin, fats, glycerol, glove powder

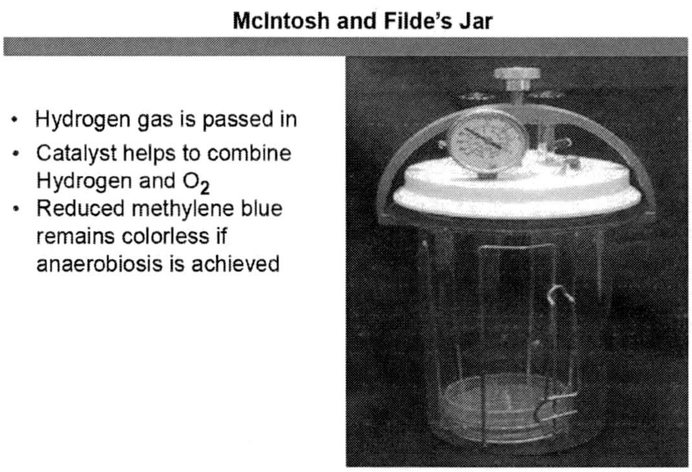

4. McIntosh and Filde's Jar

McIntosh and Filde's anaerobic jar is an instrument used in the production of an anaerobic environment (anaerobiosis)

Hydrogen gas is passed in

Catalyst helps to combine hydrogen and oxygen

The presence of air is deleterious for many anaerobic bacteria and must be incubated in its absence. The inoculated culture plates are placed inside a metal jar and the lid clamped tight. The air inside is removed using a vacuum pump. The pressure inside the chamber is reduced to 100 mm below mercury

Chapter **5**

Simple Staining

Aim: To observe the morphology of bacteria by using simple stains

Requirements: Loeffler's Methylene Blue, Dilute Carbol Fuchsin, Normal saline, Compound microscope and cedarwood oil.

Staining: Staining is an auxiliary technique used in microscopy to enhance contrast in the microscopic image. Different types of staining are Simple staining, Negative staining, Differential staining

Smear preparation:

Place one single colony of solid bacterial growth and emulsify in one drop of normal saline in the center of a clean slide. Now, with inoculating loop, mix the specimen with the saline completely and spread the mixture out to cover about half of the total slide area. Air dry it and fix it by passing over Bunsen burner. The smear is now ready for the staining procedure.

Principle:

Simple staining is performed by a watery solution of a single basic dye such as Methylene blue, Methyl violet and Basic fuschin. Positive charged cation of the basic dye combines firmely with the negatively charged radicals in the bacterial protoplasm.

The staining provides colour contrast and impart the same colour to all the bacteria. Hence it is used to see the morphology of organisms.

Procedure

- The slide is placed on the rack and is flooded with Loeffler's methylene blue/Dilute Carbol Fuchsin.
- The stain is allowed to act for 3 minutes and for 30 seconds for methylene blue and for dilute carbol fuchsin respectively.
- The slide is then washed with distilled water and gently blotted to dry.
- A drop of cedarwood oil/liquid paraffin is placed on the smear.
- The microscope is adjusted for increased light by raising the condenser, and the slide is examined with the oil immersion objective.

Preparing specimen for staining

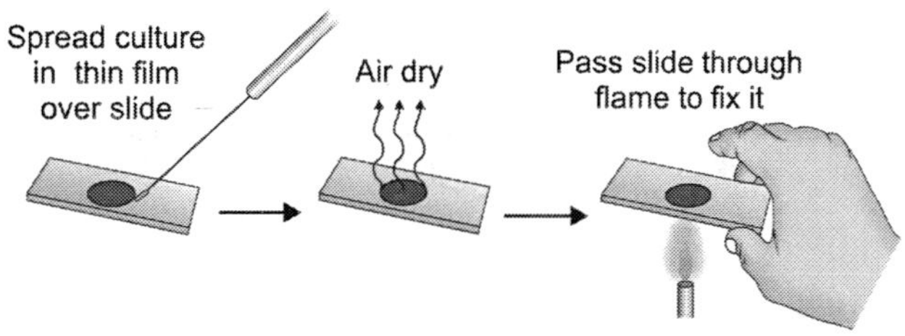

Q1. What is a stain?

Q2. What are the different methods of staining bacteria?

I. Simple staining:

a.

b.

II. Differential staining:

Negative staining:

Silver Impregnation staining :

Acid fast staining:

Albert staining

PRACTICAL 1

Stain the given smear with Loeffler's Methylene blue and record your findings with a suitable diagram.

Observation: (In terms of colour, shape and arrangement)

Inference:

PRACTICAL 2

Stain the given smear with Dilute Carbol fuchsin and record your finding with a suitable diagram.

Observation: (In terms of colour, shape and arrangement)

Inference:

Chapter 6 Gram's Staining

Aim:

To stain the given fixed smears by Gram's method.

Principle:

Certain bacteria are stained with aniline dyes, like Gentian violet .When it is subsequently treated with a solution of Iodine, mordanting action occurs. This prevents the subsequent decolorization of bacteria on treatment with acetone or alcohol. Other bacteria after similar treatment are readily decolorised.

The theories behind it are:

***pH Theory*:** Cytoplasm of gram positive bacteria is more acidic (pH2-3), hence can retain the basic dye, (pH 4-5) (crystal violet) for longer time. Iodine serves as mordant as it combines with the primary stain to form a dye-iodine complex which gets retained inside the cell.

***Cell wall theory*:** Gram positive cell has a thick peptidoglycan layer, which are tightly cross linked to each other. Peptiodoglycan, acts as a permeability barrier preventing loss of crystal violet. Alcohol ,thus shrinks the pores of thick peptidoglycan. Gram negative cell wall is more permeable , hence allowing crystal violet to flow out easily. It is so because:

The thin peptidoglycan layer in the cell wall of gram negative is not tightly cross linked.

Presence of lipopolysaccharide layer in the cell wall of gram negative bacteria, which gets disrupted easily by the action of acetone or alcohol; thus allowing the primary stain to come out of the cytoplasm.

After mordanting with Gram's iodine, bigger die-iodine complex is formed. After decolorisation, due to more lipid content in gram negative bacterial cell wall gets dissolved leading to formation of larger pores through which the dye-iodine complexes escape.

***Magnesium ribonucleate theory*:** A compound of magnesium ribonucleate and basic protein concentrated at the cell membranes helps gram positive bacteria to retain the primary dye. Gram negative bacteria do not possess this substance.

Requirements:

Gentian violet, Gram's iodine, alcohol, acetone dilute carbol fuchsin, safranine, distilled water, fixed smears, compound microscope and cedarwood oil.

Procedure

- **Primary Staining:**
  Cover the smear with Gentian violet for one minute. Gentian violet is a basic dye which combines with the acidic cytoplasm of bacterial cells.

- **Mordanting:**
  Gram's iodine is a mordant. The smear is covered with Gram's iodine for 1 minute. Gram's iodine forms a dye iodine complex.
  The cell wall of Gram positive organism is impermeable to this dye iodine complex.

- **Decolorization:**
  The slide is kept in slanting position.
  Add acetone/absolute alcohol, drop by drop till the solution which comes out of the slide is almost colorless (30 seconds)
  Gram positive organism retains primary dye (Gentian violet) while the Gram negative organisms gets decolorised.

- **Counter Staining:**
  Smear is covered with diluted carbol fuchsin/Safranine for 30 seconds and wash with water.
  Gram positive organisms remains violet, Gram negative organisms take up the counter stain and turns pink.

- Using filter paper the slide is gently blotted to dry.

- A drop of cedarwood oil/liquid paraffin is placed on the smear.

- The microscope is adjusted for increased light by raising the condenser, and the slide is examined under the oil immersion objective (100x) using the plane mirror.

Chapter 7 Morphology of Bacteria

Enumerate various bacteria based on its morphology. Draw suitable diagrams.

1. Staphylococci:

- Gram positive cocci arranged in clusters
- 1μm in size
- Cell division occurs in 3 planes
- Causes loacalized lesion and pyogenic infections

2. Streptococci:

- Gram positive cocci arranged in long chains
- 0.5–1μm in size
- Binary fission occurs in one plane
- Causes sore throat and suppurative infections

3. Pneumococci:

- Gram positive, lanceolate shaped
- Arranged in pairs (diplococci)
- Capsule is present
- Causes pneumonia

4. *Neisseria gonorrhoeae:*

- Gram negative diplococci
- Bean shaped/kidney shaped with concave adjacent sides
- Intracellular organism
- Causes sexually transmitted diseases like Gonorrhoea

5. Gram positive bacilli (*Clostrdium tetani*)

- Gram positive, slender bacilli
- Terminal spores gives it '***drumstick appearance***'
- Non-capsulated
- Motile by peritrichous flagella

6. Gram negative bacilli

- Gram negative bacilli, 1.5–3 µm in size
- Motile or non-motile
- Capsulated or non-capsulated
- Causes systemic infections

7. *Treponema pallidum*

- *T. pallidum* is a Spirochaete
- Rigid spiral forms which is actively motile , seen under dark ground microscope
- Possess Endoflagella
- Causes sexually transmitted disease-Syphilis

8. Actinomyces

- Gram positive filamentous bacteria
- Filamentous forming mycelia structure like fungi
- Form spores.
- Common cause of dental infections

Q1. Name some Gram positive organisms.

Aerobes:

Cocci:

Bacilli:

Anaerobes:

Cocci:

Bacilli:

Q2. Name some Gram negative organisms.

Aerobes:

Cocci:

Bacilli:

Anaerobes:

Cocci:

Bacilli:

Q3. Name some Coccobacilli.

Q4. What are the modifications of Gram staining.

Q5. What are the various dyes used for primary staining by Gram's technique.

Q6. What is a mordant? Name the mordant used in Gram's staining technique.

Q7. What are the various decolorising agents used in Gram's staining technique?

Q8. Name various counterstains used for Gram staining techniques.

Q9. Enumerate the differences between gram positive and gram negative cell wall.

Gram positive	Gram negative

Q10. What does the presence of pus cells indicate? What colour do they take in a Gram's stain?

Q11. What is pleomorphism? Give example.

Q12. Mention the organisms that do not possess a cell wall. What are cell wall deficient forms (CWDFs)?

Q13. How is a Gram's stain helpful in clinical practice?

- **Meningitis:**

- **Cerebral abscess:**

- **Sore throat:**

- **Respiratory tract infection:**

- **Vaginitis:**

PRACTICAL 1

Stain the given smear by Gram's technique and record your finding with a suitable diagram.

Observation: (In terms of: Colour-Gram Reaction, shape, arrangement)

Inference:

PRACTICAL 2

Stain the given smear by Gram's technique and record your finding with a suitable diagram.

Observation: (In terms of: Colour-Gram Reaction, shape, arrangement)

Inference:

Chapter 8

Hanging Drop Preparation

Aim:

To study the morphology and motility of bacteria in the given suspension.

Requirements:

A cavity slide, cover slip, vaseline, microscope and the bacterial suspension to be examined.

Procedure:

- Vaseline is applied to the four corners of a clean cover slip.
- Using a sterile loop, a loopful of the given suspension is placed on the center of the coverslip.
- A cavity slide is inverted over the cover slip so that the drop of suspension is in the centre of the cavity.
- The slide is quickly and carefully turned over so that the cover slip is on the top with the drop hanging into the cavity.
- The microscope is adjusted for reduced light by lowering the condenser.
- The edge of the drop is focussed under low power. The microscope is then turned to high power to observe the morphology and motility of the bacteria in the given suspension.

PRACTICAL 1

Prepare a Hanging Drop of the given suspension, and record your findings with a suitable diagram.

Observation:

a. Shape:

b. Motility:

Inference:

Q1. What are the various methods by which the motility of an organism can be demonstrated?

Q2. Enumerate different types of motility.

Q3. Describe the various types of flagellar arrangement found among bacteria, with suitable diagrams.

Q4. How will you differentiate true motility from Brownian/movement?

Q5. Mention

a. **Some motile bacteria:**

b. **Some non-motile bacteria:**

c. **Some bacteria that are non-motile at 37°C, but motile at 22°C:**

Q6. Describe flagella with a suitable diagram?

Q7. When do motile organisms become nonmotile?

Chapter 9 Albert's Staining

Aim: To stain the given fixed smear made from a throat swab, by Albert's technique.

Requirements: Albert's I Solution, Albert's II Solution, distilled water, fixed smears, compound microscope and cedarwood oil.

Composition of Reagents:

Albert's I Solution		**Albert's II Solution:**	
Toluidine blue	1.5 g	Iodine	6 g
Malachite green	2.0 g	Potassium iodide	9 g
Glacial acetic acid	900 mL	Distilled water	10 mL
95% Ethyl alcohol	20 mL		
Distilled water	1000 mL		

Procedure: It consists of 2 steps:

1. **Staining:**
The slide is kept covered with Albert's I solution for 3–5 minutes.
Malachite Green in Albert's I solution stains the bacilli green, while toluidine blue stains the volutin granules metachromatically, a blusih black color.

2. **Mordanting**:
The smear is covered with Albert's-II for 1 minute.
Albert's iodine acts as a mordant.

3. The slide is then washed with water and blotted to dry.
4. A drop of cedar wood oil or liquid paraffin is placed on the smear.
5. The microscope is adjusted for increased light by raising the condenser, and the smear is examined under the oil immersion objective.

PRACTICAL

The given smear is made from a throat swab. Stain by Albert's technique and record your findings with a suitable diagram.

Observation: (In terms of: colour of bacteria and granules, shape and arrangement)

Inference:

Q1. What is metachromasia?

Q2. What is the composition of metachromatic granules and what is its significance?

Q3. What is the typical arrangement of *Corynebacterium diphtheriae*? What is the reason for such an arrangement?

Q4. Mention the media used for the detection of *Corynebacteruim diphtheriae.*

Q5. Elaborate various in-vivo tests for *Corynebacterium diphtheriae.*

SUBCUTANEOUS TEST

- From overnight culture, emulsified broth prepared and 0.8 mL injected S/C into 2 guinea pigs
- One has received IM injection of 500 units of diphtheria antitoxin 18–24 hours (CONTROL)
- Unprotected guinea pig will die in 2–3 days with evidence of hemorrhage

INTRACUTANEOUS TEST

- 2 guinea pigs injected intracutaneously with 0.1 mL of emulsion broth .
- One guinea pig is protected with 500 units of antitoxin (CONTROL)
- Other guinea pig injected with 50 units of antitoxin intraperitoneally.
- If strain is virulent, inflammation occurs at the site of injection—leading to necrosis in 48–72 hours in test animal. No animal dies in this test

Q6. Elaborate various in-vitro tests for *Corynebacterium diphtheriae*

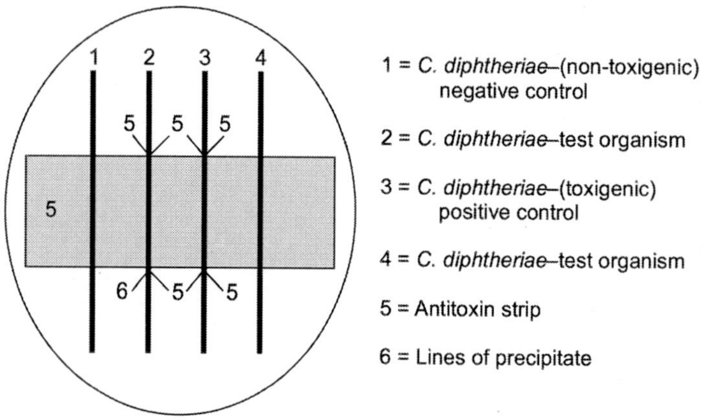

- Immunodiffusion test
- A rectangular strip soaked with 100 units/ml of Diphtheria antitoxin is placed on Horse serum agar plate (medium in fluid state).
- Test strain streaked when agar solidifies at right angle along with positive and negative controls.
- Incubate at 37°C for 48 hours
- Toxin produced by bacterial growth diffuses in agar and produces a line of precipitation where it meets the antitoxin at optimum conc.
- No ppt line on non-toxigenic strain

Q7. What are the complications of diphtheria?

Q8. How can diphtheria be prevented?

Chapter **10**

Ziehl Neelsen's Staining

Aim: To stain the given fixed smear of sputum by Ziehl Neelsen's technique for detection of Mycobacterium.

Principle: Ordinary aniline dye solutions do not readily penetrate the substance of the tubercle bacilli and therefore it is not suitable for staining. By the use of powerful staining solution that contains phenol and with the application of heat, which act as a mordant, it can be made to penetrate the bacillus. Once stained the tubercle bacillus will withstand the action of powerful decolorizing agents, thus retains the stain .

Requirements: Strong Carbol fuchsin, 20–25% H_2SO_4, 95% alcohol or acid alcohol, Methylene blue solution, distilled water, spirit lamp, compound microscope and cedarwood oil/liquid paraffin.

Composition of strong carbol fuchsin:

Basic Fuchsin	- 5 gms.
Absolute Alcohol	- 50 ml.
Phenol (crystalline)	- 25 gm
Distiled water	- 500 ml

Procedure

Primary staining and mordanting:

The fixed smear is flooded with strong Carbol fuchsin for 5 minute and heated intermittently. Until the steam rises, taking care to see that the stain does not boil and smear does not get charred. Smear is then washed well with distilled water.

The basic fuchsin in strong Carbol fuchsin is a basic stain, while carbolic acid acts as a mordant. On heating, the mycolic acid in the cell wall of the acid fast organisms is liquefied and the basic stain imbibed by the organism is fixed by the mordant.

- **Decolorisation**:

  The slide is then covered with 20–25% H_2SO_4 for 2–3 mins and washed with water. This step is repeated till the smear becomes colourless. With this, only acid fast organisms retain the basic stain, while the cells and other organisms are rendered colourless.

  Decolourise it with 95% alcohol or acid alcohol. Decolourising with alcohol; saprophytes can be differentiated from Mycobacterium tuberculosis, as saprophytes are only acid fast whereas Mycobacterium tubercle bacilli is acid as well as alcohol fast.
- **Counter Staining:**

  The slide is covered with methylene blue or 1–2 minutes, washed with water and blotted to dry.

  Acid fast organisms remain pink while the other organisms and cells, take up the counter stain and turn blue.
- A drop of cedarwood oil or liquid paraffin is placed on the stained smear.
- The microscope is adjusted for increased light by raising the condenser and the smear is examined under the oil immersion objective using the plane mirror.

RNTCP Grading

Ziehl-Neelsen Staining Grading			
Finding	***No. of fields***	***Grading***	***Result***
No AFB in 100 oil immersion field	**100**	**0**	**Neg**
1-9 AFB per 100 oil immersion field	**100**	**scanty**	**Pos**
10–99 AFB per 100 oil immersion fields	**100**	**1+**	**Pos**
1-10 AFB per oil immersion field	**50**	**2+**	**Pos**
>10 AFB per oil immersion field	**20**	**3+**	**Pos**

Q1. Mention some acid fast organisms/structure.

Q2. What are the various specimens obtained in the laboratory for the diagnosis of tuberculosis?

Q3. Name the various media used for the isolation of *Mycobacterium tuberculosis.*

Q4. Mention the techniques used to concentrate mycobacteria in clinical specimens. When are they indicated?

Q5. Describe Petroff's method.

Q6. What is Koch's phenomenon?

Q7. What is Mantoux test?

Q8. What is B.C.G.? How is it useful?

Q9. What are the differences between *Mycobacterium tuberculosis* and *Mycobacterium leprae*?

a.	**Morphology**	:	
b.	**Staining technique**	:	
c.	**Generation time**	:	
d.	**Culture**	:	
e.	**Laboratory animals used**	:	

Q.10. What are the differences between Human and Bovine tubercle bacilli

Q.11 What are the various concentrations of H_2SO_4 used for various Mycobacteria.

Q.12 What is Kinyuon staining.

PRACTICAL 1

Stain the given smear of sputum by Ziehl Nelsen's technique and record your findings with a suitable diagram.

Observation: (In terms of: colour, shape, arrangement and background)

Inference:

PRACTICAL

Stain the given smear of sputum by Ziehl Nelsen's technique and record your findings with a suitable diagram.

Observation: (In terms of: colour, shape, arrangement and background)

Inference:

PRACTICAL

Stain the given smear of sputum by Ziehl Nelsen's technique and record your findings with a suitable diagram.

Observation: (In terms of: colour, shape, arrangement and background)

Inference:

PRACTICAL

Stain the given smear of sputum by Ziehl Nelsen's technique and record your findings with a suitable diagram.

Observation: (In terms of: colour, shape, arrangement and background)

Inference:

Chapter **11**

Culture Media and Culture Methods

Definition:

Culture media are required to grow the organism from the infected material to identify the causative pathogen. Basic constituents of soild culture media are:

- Water - Source of hydrogen and oxygen
- Electrolyte - Sodium chloride or other electrolytes
- Peptone - Complex mixture of partially digested proteins
- Meat extract - Contains protein degradation products, inorganic salts, carbohydrates and growth factors
- **Agar Agar - Prepared from sea weed (*Algae-geladium spp.*). Used in conc. of *2-3%*. It melts at 98°C and solidifies at 42°C. It is an inert substance, neither stimulate nor it inherit the growth**
- Blood or serum - Used for enriching culture media. 5–10% sheep blood is used for enriched media to provide extra nutrition to fastidious organisms.

Classification of Media:

1. Based on physical state

- Liquid media
- Semi-solid media
- Solid media

2. Based on presence of molecular oxygen and reducing substances

- Aerobic media
- Anaerobic media

3. Based on nutritional factors

a. Simple media
b. Complex media
c. Synthetic media
d. Special media
   - Enriched media
   - Enrichment media
   - Selective media
   - Differential media
   - Indicator media
   - Transport media

I. CULTIVATION OF AEROBIC BACTERIA

1. Culture Media (Aerobic)

Solid Media: Dispensed in petri dishes/McCartney bottles.

Type of medium	*Name of medium*	Composition	Laboratory use
A. Simple	*Nutrient agar*	Peptone + Meat extract + Agar + NaCl	Culture and demonstration of pigmentation of different bacteria
B. Complex/Special a. Differential	*MacConkey's agar*	Lactose + Peptone + NaCl + Bile salts + Neutral red + Agar	Differentiate between lactose and non-lactose fermenters
b. Enriched	*1. Blood agar*	Nutrient agar + 5% Sheep blood	Differentiate between hemolytic and non-hemolytic bacteria
	2. Chocolate agar	Blood agar heated at 75°C for 10–15 mins leads to release of X and V factors	H. influenzae, Neisseria
	3. Loffler's serum slope	Nutrient broth + glucose + horse serum	Coynebacterium diphtheriae

c. Selective	***1. Thayer-Martin mediun***	**Agar base + Hb + growth factor + antibiotics like Vancomycin, Colistin + Nystatin**	**Isolation of *Neisseria gonorrhoeae***
	2. Potassium tellurite agar	**Blood agar + potassium tellurite**	**For *Corynebacterium diphtheriae***
	3. Wilson and Blair Medium	**Nutrient agar + glucose phosphate + brilliant green + bismuth sulphate**	**Isolation of *Salmonella* spp.**
	4. Deoxycholate citrate agar (DCA)	**Peptone + Lactose + Sodium deoxycholate + sodium citrate+ neutral red**	**Isolation of *Salmonella* and *Shigella***
	5. TCBS medium (thiosulphate citrate bile salt sucrose agar)	**Peptone + sodium thiosulphate + sodium citrate + NaCl+ sucrose + ox bile + bromothymol blue**	**Isolation of *Vibrio cholerae***
	6. Lowenstein Jensen medium	**Egg + glycerol + NaCl+ malachite green**	**Isolation of *Mycobacteria tubercle***
	7. Muller Hinton agar	**Beef extract + casein hydrosylate + starch**	**For antibiotic susceptibility testing**

Transport media: It is devised to maintain the viability of a pathogen and to avoid overgrowth of other containments during transit of sample from patient to laboratory. It is available as sterile disposable swab kits.

Name of the medium	*Composition*	*Laboratory use*
Stuart transport medium	**Sodium thioglycolate + sodium glycerophosphate + calcium chloride + agar + methylene blue + distilled water**	**For maintaining the viability of *Neisseria* gonococci on swab**
Amie's transport medium	**Sodium thioglycolate + NaCl+ KCl + $CaCl_2$+ disodium hydrogen phosphate +potassium dihydrogn phosphate + charcoal + agar + distilled water**	**For maintaining the viability of *Neisseria* gonococci on swab**
Pike's medium	**Blood agar containing crystal violet + sodium azide**	**For *Strep. pyogenes, H. influenzae* swabs**
Glycerol saline transport medium	**Glycerol + NaCl + disodium hydrogen phosphate + phenol red 0.02%+ water**	**For *Salmonella typhi* feces culture**
Venkat Ramakrishna medium	**Crude sea salt + peptone + distilled water at pH- 8.6-8.9**	**For *Vibrio cholerae***
Viral transport medium (VTM)	**Modified Hank›s Balanced Salt Solution supplemented with bovine serum albumin, sucrose, glutamic acid, and gelatin.**	**For transporting H1N1 virus**

Liquid Media: Dispensed in tubes:

Type of medium	*Name of medium*	*Composition*	*Laboratory use*
A Basal	***1. Peptone medium***	**Peptone + NaCl + water**	**For sugar fermentation test**
B Special **a. Enriched:**	***1. Glucose broth***	**Nutrient broth + glucose**	**For *Streptococcus***
	2. Hiss Serum	**Serum+ peptone water**	**For *Corynebacterium***
b. Enrichment:	***1. Selenite F broth***	**Peptone water + sodium selenite**	**Isolation of *Salmonella* and *Shigella***
i. For specimens other than blood:	***2. Tetrathionate broth***	**Nutrient broth + sodium thiosulbate, + calcium carbonate + iodine solution**	**For *Salmonella***
	3. Alkaline peptone water	**Peptone water pH = 8.6**	**For *Vibrio cholerae***
Liquid media used for blood culture:	***1. Brain heart infusion broth***	**Nutrient broth + dehydrated heart meat**	**Blood culture**
	2. Liver Infusion broth	**Nutrient broth + crushed lean liver of sheep**	**Blood culture of pyogenic bacteria and enteric bacilli**
	3. Glucose broth	**Nutrient broth + glucose**	**For pyogenic organism**
	4. Bile broth	**Nutrient broth + bile**	**For *Salmonella***

Biphasic media: Dispensed in blood culture bottles.

Name of medium	*Composition*	*Laboratory use*
Casteneda medium	***Brain heart infusion broth and agar***	For blood culture for Brucellosis

II. CULTIVATION OF ANAEROBIC BACTERIA

1. Culture Media (Anaerobic):

S. No.	*Type of medium*	*Name of Medium*	*Composition*	*Laboratory use*
1.	**Liquid medium**	***Robertson Cooked Medium***	Nutrient broth + Minced meat	Growth of anaerobic bacteria
		Thiogylcolate medium	Nutrient broth + 1% thioglycolate + Reasuzurin	Growth of anaerobic bacteria

2. Inoculation Methods

Inoculation is done with a loop made of Nichrome wire of 24 S. W. G size. The loop 2–4 mm. In diameter with a wire 2 to 3" long and is sterilized in the Bunsen flame.

Various methods of inoculation are employed:

S. No.	Name of method	Diagram	Procedure	Indication
1.	**Streak culture**		Loop is sterilized on flame and inoculum is taken and smeared on a well. From there create a parallel streaks A,B,C and the tail	To get isolated colonies
2.	**Lawn culture**		Hooding the plate with liquid culture suspension	For antibiotic sensitivity pattern
3.	**Stroke culture**		Streaking on a nutrient agar slope	Demonstration of gel liquefaction and oxygen requirements of bacteria
4.	**Pour plate method**		Serial dilutions of bacteria onto molten agar	Bacterial count and quantitative anaylsis of urine

Q1. How are bacteria categorised on the basis of their oxygen and temperature requirement?

On basis of their oxygen requirement

- **Obligate aerobes:** Those bacteria which require only oxygen for their growth, e.g. *Pseudomonas aeruginosa*
- **Facultative anaerobes:** Aerobes but can also grow without oxygen
- **Microaerophilic:** It can grow in presence of traces of oxygen, e.g. *Campylobacter jejuni. H. pylori*
- **Anaerobes:** Obligate or strict anaerobes can grow only in the absence of oxygen, e.g. *Clostridium tetani*
- **Capnophilic:** Some bacteria require 5–10% higher amount of carbon dioxide for their growth, e.g. *Brucella abortus*

On basis of their temperature

Mainly bacteria grow at 37°C. Bacteria are further grouped as:

- **Mesophiles:** Grows at temp between 25°C and 40°C e.g. all pathogenic bacteria
- **Psychrophiles:** Grows at temp. below 20°C. e g. Soil and water saprophytes
- **Thermophiles:** Grows at temp. Between 55°C and 80°C e.g. Bacillus stearothermophilus

Q2. What is agar agar? What percentage is used in Media preparation?

Q3. Give example of Lactose fermenters and Non-Lactose fermenters.

Q4. Mention the indications of blood culture.

Chapter 12 Identification of Bacteria by Biochemical Reactions

1. CATALASE TEST

Principle: The enzyme catalase decomposes hydrogen peroxide (H_2O_2) into water and nascent oxygen. The presence of enzyme in a bacterial isolates is evident when a small inoculum is introduced into H_2O_2 and the rapid elaboration of oxygen bubbles occurs. The lack of catalase enzyme is evident by a lack of or weak bubble.

Procedure: With an inoculating needle or a wooden applicator stick, transfer growth from the centre of a colony to the surface of a glass slide. Add a drop of of 3% hydrogen peroxide and observe the bubble formation. This test is used to differentiate *Staphylococcus* spp. and *Streptococcus* spp.

Interpretation: The rapid and sustained production of bubbles or effervescence constitutes a positive test because of the production of enzyme catalase.

Quality Control

Positive control: *Staphylococcus aureus*
Negative control: *Streptococcus pyogenes*

2. OXIDASE TEST

Principle: Cytochromes are iron-containing hemoproteins that act as the last link in the chain of aerobic respiration by transferring electrons(hydrogen) to oxygen, with formation of water. The cytochrome system is found in aerobic, microaerophilic and facultatively anaerobic organisms. The dye 1% solution of tetra methyl-para-phenylene-diamine dihydrochloride is oxidized to indophenol blue producing deep purple colour.

Procedure: Wet filter paper method is used in this test. Strips of Whatmann's No. 1 filter paper is soaked with a little freshly made 1% solution of tetra methyl-para-phenylene-diamine dihydrochloride and then with a help of sterile glass rod a single colony from the medium is rubbed over the strip.

Interpretation: A positive reaction is indicated by an intense deep purple blue color appearing within 5–10 seconds and a negative reaction by absence of coloration or by coloration later than 60 seconds.

Quality Control

Positive control: *Pseudomonas aeruginosa* ATCC 27583
Negative control: *Escherichia coli* ATCC 25922

3. COAGULASE TEST

This test is done to differentiate between *Staphylococcus* species. Both slide and tube coagulase test is done.

Slide Coagulase Test

Principle:
Slide coagulase test detects bound coagulase which is attached to the bacterial cell wall and is not present in culture filtrate. Fibrin strands are formed between the bacterial cells when suspended in plasma (fibrinogen), causing them to clump not visible aggregates.

Procedure:
A smooth milky suspension of the growth is made in normal saline over a clean glass slide. Make similar suspension of control positive and negative strains to confirm the proper reactivity of the plasma. To the test suspension a loop full of undiluted human plasma is added and the suspension is observed for the appearance of coarse clumps.

Interpretation:
It is read as positive when a coarse clumping of cocci is visible to the naked eye within 10 seconds. Negative is read when there is absence of clumping .

Tube Coagulase Test

Principle:
Coagulase is a protein that has prothrombin like activity which can convert fibrinogen to fibrin. A visible clot is seen. Heat labile protein secreted free into the medium and clots the rapid plasma in presence of factor known as Coagulase Reactive Factor (CRF), which is similar to prothrombin present in plasma and converts fibrinogen into fibrin.

Free coagulase + CRF ⟶ CRF Coagulase

Fibrinogen ⟶ Fibrin

Quality Control
Positive control: *Staphylococcus aureus*
Negative control: *Staphylococcus epidermidis*

4. INDOLE TEST

Principle:
This test is done to demonstrate the ability of certain bacteria that possess enzyme tryptophanase , which are capable of hydrolysing and deamining tryptophan with the production of indole, pyruvic acid and ammonia. Indole, a benzyl pyrrole, is one of the metabolic degradation products of amino acid tryptophan

Procedure:

Kovac's reagent method is employed. Kovac's reagent preparation

Amyl or isoamyl alcohol	-	150 mL
p-dimethylaminobenzaldehyde	-	10 g
Concentrated HCl	-	50 mL

Individual colonies are inoculated on to peptone water and incubated at 37°C for 18–24 hrs. To this 0.5 mL of Kovac's reagent is added and gently shaken.

Interpretation: Appearance of bright fuschia pink colored ring at the interface of reagent and the broth within seconds after adding the reagent is indicative of the presence of indole and is a positive test.

Quality Control
Positive control: *Escherichia coli* ATCC 25922
Negative control: *Klebsiella pneumoniae.*

5. UREASE TEST

Principle:
Urease is an enzyme possessed by many species of microorganisms. This test is done to determine the ability of bacteria to decompose urea into ammonia. Christensen's urea agar medium is used. Indicator used is Phenol red

Procedure:

Inoculate heavily over the entire surface of Christensen's urea agar medium with the peptone water culture and incubate at 37°C. Examine after 4hrs and then overnight incubation.

Interpretation

Positive: When the indicator turned to pink-purple.

Negative: No change in color.

Quality Control
Positive control: *Proteus* species
Negative control: *Escherichia coli*

6. CITRATE UTILIZATION TEST

Principle:

The utilization of citrate by a test bacterium is detected in a citrate medium by the production of alkaline by products. To determine the ability of certain bacteria to obtain energy in a manner by utilizing citrate as a sole source of carbon for its growth. Simmons citrate medium is used to know the utilization of citrate. Indicator is bromothymol blue

Procedure:

The citrate slant is inoculated with the suspected single colony and medium is incubated at 37°C for 24 to 48 hrs. A positive reaction is indicated by the blue color and streak of growth. A negative reaction if original green color persists and no growth along the streak line.

Quality Control

Positive control: *Enterobacter aerogenes*

Negative control: *Escherichia coli*

7. TRIPLE SUGAR IRON AGAR TEST

Principle:

This is done to determine ability of bacteria to ferment carbohydrates incorporated in a growth medium and production of hydrogen sulphide. Triple sugar iron (TSI) agar medium contains 10 parts lactose, 10 parts sucrose, 1 part glucose and peptone.Phenol red and ferrous sulphate serve as indicator of acidification and H_2S production respectively. With a sterile straight inoculating wire, touch the top of a well with isolated colony.

Procedure:

Inoculate TSI slant by first stabbing through the centre of the medium to the bottom of the tube and then streaking the surface of the agar slant. Incubate the tube at 37°C for 18-24 hrs. The result is interpreted as follows:

Interpretation:

Slant /butt	*Colour*	*Utilization*
Alkaline slant/Acid butt(K/A)	Red/Yellow	Glucose only fermented; peptone is utilized
Acid slant/acid butt (A/A)	Yellow/Yellow	Glucose fermented, lactose and or sucrose fermented
Alkaline butt/Alkaline butt (K/K)	Red/Red	No fermentation of glucose, lactose or sucrose.

A black precipitate in the butt indicates production of ferrous sulphide and H_2S gas. Bubbles or cracks in the media indicate the production of CO_2 or H_2.

8. METHYL RED TEST

Principle:

Methyl red is quantitative test for production of acid, requiring positive organism to produce strong acids (lactic acid, acetic acid, formic acid) from glucose through the mixed acid fermentation pathway. This test is to determine the ability of bacteria which can maintain the low pH after prolonged incubation.

Procedure:

Inoculate the glucose phosphate broth with a pure culture of test organism and incubate at 37°C for 48 hrs (no fewer than 48 hrs). To this, add about five drops of the methyl red reagent. Mix and read immediately.

Interpretation:

Development of stable red color in the surface of medium indicates sufficient acid production to lower pH to 4.4 and constitutes a positive test.

Quality control:

Positive control: *Escherichia coli*
Negative control: *Enterobacter aerogenes*

9. VOGES PROSKAUER TEST

Principle:

Pyruvic acid is a pivotal compound formed in the fermentative degradation of glucose, further metabolized through various metabolic pathways, depending upon the enzyme systems possessed by different bacteria, where the end product is acetoin (acetyl methyl carbinol). In the presence of atmospheric oxygen and 40% potassium hydroxide, acetoin is converted into diacetyl and alpha-naphthol serves as a catalyst to bring out a red complex.

Procedure:

Inoculate the glucose phosphate peptone broth with a pure culture of test organism and incubate at 37°C for 48 hours. To this add 0.6 mL of 5% α-naphthol followed by 0.2 mL of 40% potassium hydroxide. Shake the tube gently to expose the medium to atmospheric oxygen and allow to remain it undisturbed for 10–15 minutes.

Interpretation:

A positive reaction is indicated by the development of a red colour in 15 mins,indicating the presence of diacetyl, the oxidation product of acetoin. It turns crimson red in color in 30 minutes.

Quality Control

Positive control: *Enterobacter aerogenes*
Negative control: *Escherichia coli*

10. SUGAR FERMENTATION TEST

Principle:

This test is done to determine the ability of an organism to ferment a specific carbohydrate that is incorporated in a basal medium, thereby producing acid with or without visible gas.

Procedure:

The test is performed on conventional culture media with test sugars. The common sugar fermentation media used for present study were glucose, lactose, sucrose, maltose, mannose, arabinose and xylose. From the peptone water tube (Which was incubated for 2 hrs. after inoculation) all the sugar fermentation media are inoculated with the help of a Pasteur pipette. After the different media are inoculated, these are incubated at 37°C for 18–24 hrs. After 24 hrs the sugar media are examined for the production of acid indicated by pink colour and gas (presence of an air bubble inside the Durham's tube).

Interpretation:

Positive test is indicated by change in color to pink with or without gas formation in Durham's tube. Negative test is indicated by growth, but no change in color.

11. OXIDATION/FERMENTATION TEST (MODIFIED HUGH AND LEIFSON)

Principle:

This test is done to know where the organism uses carbohydrate substrate to produce acid by products either oxidatively or fermentatively.

Procedure:

Hugh-Leifson basal medium is prepared and carbohydrate to be added is sterilised separately and added to give final concentration of 1%. The medium is then tubed to a depth of about 4 cm.
Duplicate tubes of medium were inoculated by stabbing. One tube is promptly covered with liquid paraffin to a depth of 1 cm and is incubated at 37°C for 18–24 hrs.

Interpretation:

Acid production is detected in the medium by the appearance of a yellow color. In the case of oxidative organisms, colour production may be first noted near the surface of medium.

Following are reaction patterns:

Open tube	***Covered tube***	***Metabolism***
Acid (yellow)	Alkaline (green)	Oxidative
Acid (yellow)	Acid (yellow)	Fermentative
Alkaline (green or blue)	Alkaline (green or blue)	Non-saccharolytic

12. NITRATE REDUCTION TEST

Principle:

The test is used to determine the ability of an organism to reduce nitrate to nitrites which is used for the identification of mainly Enterobacteriaceae. The reduction of nitrate to nitrite is determined by adding sulfanilic acid and alpha-naphthylamine. The sulfanilic acid and nitrate forms a diazonium salt. The diazonium salt then couples with α-naphthylamine to produce a red, water soluble azo dye.

Procedure:

This liquid medium is inoculated with the suspected single colony and the medium is incubated for 18–24 hours.

Add 0.1 mL of the test reagent to the test culture. The test reagent is prepared by mixing equal volumes of solution A (8.0 g of sulfanilic acid in 1 L of acetic acid 5 mol/L) and solution B (5.0 g of α-naphtylamine in 1 L of acetic acid 5 mol/L).

Interpretation:

Development of red color within 30 seconds after adding the test reagents indicates the presence of nitrites and represents a positive reaction for nitrate reduction.

Quality Control

Positive control: *Escherichia coli*

Negative control: *Acinetobacter baumannii*

13. PHENYLALANINE DEAMINASE TEST (PPA)

Principle:

To determine the ability of bacteria to deaminate phenylalanine to phenyl pyruvic acid. Of the Enterobacteriaceae, only members of the *Proteus, Morganella* and *Providencia* genera possess the deaminase enzyme.

Procedure:

This test was done to know the ability of the organism to deaminate phenylalanine with the production of phenyl pyruvic acid, which reacts with ferric salts to give green color. Inoculate it with pure growth and incubate 37°C for 18–24 hrs. After incubation, allow a few drops of 10% solution of ferric chloride to run over the growth on the slope.

Interpretation:

The immediate appearance of an intense green color indicates the presence of phenylpyruvic acid and a positive test.

Quality Control

Positive control: *Proteus* species

Negative control: *Escherichia coli*

14. AMINO ACID DECARBOXYLASES

Principle:

Decarboxylases are group of substrate specific enzymes that are capable of reacting with the carboxyl portion of amino acids, forming alkaline-reacting amines. The conversion of arginine to citrulline is a dehydrolase, in which an NH_2 group is removed from arginine. Citrulline is next converted to ornithine, which then undergoes decarboxylation to form putrescine.

Procedure:

Two Moller decarboxylases broth base is used. The amino acid to be tested is added to the decarboxylase base before inoculation with the test organism. A control tube, consisting only the base without the amino acid, must also be set up in parallel. Both tubes are anerobically incubated by overlaying the mineral oil. Incubate at 37°C for 18–24 hours. At initial stages of incubation, both the tubes turn yellow, owing to the fermentation of small, amount of glucose in the medium. If amino acid is decarboxylated, alkaline amines are formed and the medium reverts to original purple colour. Indicators are cresol red and bromocresol purple

L-lysine ———— lysine decarboxylase ————→ cadaverine + carbondioxide

Bromocresol purple ———— cadaverine ————→ bromocresol purple

(yellow) (lavender purple)

Interpretation

Conversion of the control tube to a yellow color indicates that the organism is viable and that the pH of the medium has been lowered sufficiently to activate the decarboylase enzymes. Reversion of the tube containing the amino acid to a blue-purple color indicates a positive test owing to the formation of amines from the decarboxylation reaction.

Quality Control

Amino acid	*Positive control*	*Negative control*
Lysine	Enterobacter aerrogenes	Enterobacter cloacae
Ornithine	Enterobacter cloacae	Klebsiella pneumoniae
Arginine	Enterobacter cloacae	Enterobacter aerogenes

Chapter 13

Principles and Uses of Antimicrobial Agents

All strains of bacteria are not alike in their susceptibility to antimicrobial drugs. Therefore, the reliable guide to the therapeutic use of antimicrobial agents is an in vitro sensitivity test. Two methods are generally in use:

1. **Dilution test:** Serial dilutions of the drug in broth or agar are inoculated with the test organism and incubated overnight. The lowest concentration of the drug. i.e., the highest dilution in which the organism does not show growth, is considered as the minimal inhibitory concentration (MIC) of the drug for the particular strain.

2. **Disc diffusion test:** Six mm discs made out of What man filter paper are impregnated with antibiotics and preserved at 4°C in a refrigerator. The discs are impregnated with a standard quantity of the drugs. The medium used is Mueller Hinton Agar on which a lawn culture is done and individual discs are placed. The plates are incubated overnight and inhibition of growth of the organism to each drug is estimated.

The Disc diffusion test can be done by two methods:

A. Stoke's method: The zones of inhibition of the test organism are compared directly with those of the control stain of standard sensitivity, inoculated on the same plate.

B. Kirby-Bauer's method: The zones of inhibition of the test organism are compared with critical zone diameters given in a previously prepared scale. The scale correlates zone size with the MIC.

- The blood concentration achieved by the dose of anti-microbial prescribed, should be higher than MIC, but should not be toxic to the patient.

PRACTICAL 1

Record the drug sensitivity of the organism demonstrated, using Kirby-Bauer method.

The given organism is:

Sensitive to

Resistant to

Q1. What are bactericidal and bacteriostatic drugs?

Q2. When Penicillin and Cephalosporin are indicated? How do they work?

Q3. Name the antibiotics which acts via different mechanism.

a. **Cell wall inhibitors**

b. **Protein synthesis inhibitors**

c. **Ribosomes**

Q4. Tabulate the differences between mutational and transferable drug resistance.

Chapter 14 Collection and Transport of Clinical Specimens and Various Clinical Syndromes

- **CEREBROSPINAL FLUID**

  Technique of Collection:

  Processing:

- **THROAT SWAB**

  Technique of Collection:

  Processing:

- **SPUTUM**

  Technique of Collection:

  Processing:

- **PUS**

  Technique of Collection:

  Processing:

- **VAGINAL SWAB**

  Technique of Collection:

  Processing:

- **URINE**

  Technique of Collection:

  Processing:

- **STOOL**

  Technique of Collection:

  Processing:

- **BLOOD**

  Technique of Collection:

  Processing:

Q1. Define P.U.O. Enumerate various causes and write the laboratory diagnosis for it.

Definition: Any febrile illness with a body temperature more than 38°C or more than 100°F, lasting for more than 3 weeks or longer, without any obvious cause or remain uncertain in spite of investigations.

Causes:

Bacterial

Localised pyogenic infections:	*Systemic bacterial infections:*
Appendicitis	Mycobacterial infections
Cholangitis	Typhoid fever
Cholecystitis	Mycoplasma
Localised abscess	Chlamydial infections
Mesentric lymphadenitis	Brucellosis
Osteomyelitis	Meliodosis
Pelvic inflammatory disease	Listeriosis
Sinusitis	Bartonellosis
Suppurative throbophlebitis	Spirocheate infections
Intravascular infections	

Viral: Chikungunya fever, Dengue fever, Cytomegalovirus and EBV infection, Coxsackie group B, Viral hepatitis, HIV infection

Fungal: Aspergillosis, Mucormycosis, Blastomycosis, Histoplasmosis, Coccidioidomycosis, Paracoccidioidomycosis, Candidiasis, Cryptococcosis, Pneumocystis infection, Sporotrichosis

Parasitic: Malaria, Amoebiasis, Leishmaniasis, Chagas' disease, Toxoplasmosis, Strongyloidiasis

Q2. Mention the various organisms causing Meningitis. Enumerate its lab diagnosis

Definiton: Meningitis is an inflammation of the meninges surrounding the brain and spinal cord, which implies to infection of subarachnoid space or leptomeninges.

Types of meningitis: Based on leukocytes in CSF, it is grouped into

1. ***Pyogenic meningitis*:** Characterised by elevated polymorphonuclear cells in CSF

   Causes of pyogenic meningitis are:
   - Neonates or Infants of 0–2 months-*Escherichia coli,* Group B *Streptococcus, Klebsiella pneumoniae, Listeria monocytogenes*
   - 2–20 yrs- *Neisseria meningitides, Haemophilus influenzae, Streptococcus pneumoniae*
   - >20 yrs- *Streptococcus pneumoniae, Haemophilus influenzae* and *Neisseria meningitidis*

2. ***Aseptic meningitis:*** Characterised by elevated lymphocytes in CSF.

   Causes of aseptic meningitis are:

Bacteria: *M. tuberculosis, Treponema pallidum, Leptospira*

Fungi: *Cryptococcus neoformans*

Virus: Enterovirus, Herpes Simplex virus 1 and 2, Varicella zoster virus, Cytomegalovirus, Epstein Barr virus, Mumps virus, Arbovirus, Adenovirus, Rubella virus and HIV

Parasite: *Naegleria fowleri, Acanthamoeba* spp., *Toxoplasma gondii*

Q3. Mention the various organisms causing pneumonia.

Definition: Pneumonia refers to inflammation of lungs which can be classified as:

A. ***Community acquired:*** Patients acquire organisms from community.

   Bacterial causes: *Streptococcus pneumoniae, Mycoplasma pneumoniae, Haemophilus influenzae, Chlamydophila pneumoniae.*
   Viral Causes: Influenza virus, adenovirus, respiratory syncytial virus, parainfluenza virus.

B. ***Hospital acquired:*** Patients acquire organisms in hospital setting.

   Bacterial causes: *Streptococcus pneumoniae, Mycoplasma pneumoniae, Haemophilus influenzae, Chlamydophila pneumoniae, Legionella pneumoniae, Staphylococcus aureus,* Gram negative bacilli.
   Viral causes: Influenza virus, adenovirus, respiratory syncytial virus, parainfluenza virus.

Q4. Mention the various organisms causing sore throat

Bacterial: *Streptococcus pyogenes (most common), Streptococcus pneumoniae, Corynebacterium diphtheria, Corynebacterium ulcerans, Treponema vincentii, Leptotrichia buccalis, Arachanobacterium* spp.

Fungal: *Candida albicans*

Viral: Influenza virus, parainfluenza virus, coxsackie virus, rhinovirus, coronavirus, Epstein-Barr virus, adenovirus

Q5. What are the various causative agents of Urinary tract infection? What is Kass criteria? Write the laboratory diagnosis for UTI.

Definition: Urinary tract infection is defined as disease caused by microbial invasion of the urinary tract that extends from renal cortex of kidney to urethral meatus.

UTI is classified into two types:

Upper UTI: Involves kidney and ureter.

Lower UTI: Involves urethra and bladder

Causes:

Bacteria: Gram negative - *Escherichia coli, Klebsiella pneumoniae, Proteus mirabilis, Pseudomonas aeruginosa, Acinetobacter* spp., *Enterobacter* spp., *Serratia* spp.

Gram positive cocci : *Staphyloococcus saprophyticus, Staphylococcus aureus, Staphylococcus epidermidis, Enterococcus* spp.

Viral: Herpes simplex virus, adenovirus, JC and BK virus, cytomegalovirus.

Fungal: *Candida albicans.*

Parasitic: *Schistosoma haematobium, Trichomonas vaginalis*

Kass Criteria (Significant Bacteriuria):

Presence of bacteria more than 10^5 CFU/ml in a mid stream urine sample by standard loop technique on Blood agar/ CLED agar. It indicates active infection

Q6. Mention the various organisms causing sexually transmitted diseases. Write the laboratory diagnosis for STDs.

Definition: STDs are group of communicable diseases which are transmitted predominantly or entitely by sexual contact and caused by bacteria, virus, protozoa and fungus.

Classification based on clinical manifestations:

Painless genital ulcer:

- Syphlis: *Treponema pallidum*
- Lymphogranuloma venereum: *Chlamydia trachomatis*
- Donovonasis: *Klebsiella granulomatis*

Painful genital ulcer:

Chancroid: *Haemophilus ducreyi*
Herpes genitalis: HSV1 and 2

Uretheral Discharge

- Gonorrhoea: *Neisseria gonorrhoeae*
- Non-gonococcal urethritis—*Chlamydia trachomatis, Ureaplasma urealyticum, Mycoplama genitalium, Mycoplasma hominis*, Herpes Simplex virus, *Candida albicans, Trichomonas vaginalis.*

Vaginal Discharge

Vulvovaginal candidiasis: *Candida albicans*, non-albicans *Candida*
Bacterial vaginosis: *Gardnerall vaginalis, Mobilincus* spp.
Trichomonas vaginitis: *Trichomonas vaginalis*

Genital Wart

Human papilloma virus.

Systemic Manifestations

Pelvic inflammatory disease: *N. gonorrhoeae* and *C. trachomatis*
No genital lesions: HIV, HBV, HCV.

Q.7 Enumerate various causes of diarrhea and dysentry and what is their lab diagnosis?

DIARRHOEA: As per WHO, diarrhea is defined as passage of three or more loose or liquid stools per day, in excess than the usual habitat for that person.

Causes are:
Bacteria (Enterotoxin mediated): *Vibrio cholerae, Vibrio parahemolyticus, Escherichia coli* (Enterotoxigenic), *Clostridium perfringes, Aeromonas* spp.

Cytotoxin mediated: *Shigella* spp., Enterohemorrhagic *E.coli, Yersinia enterocolitica, Listeria monocytogenes, Clostridum difficle.*

Neurotoxin mediated: *Staphylococcus aureus, Bacillus cereus, Clostridium botulinum.*

Viral: Rotavirus, Norovirus, Astrovirus, Calcivirus, Norwalk virus.

Parasite: *Giardia lamblia, Cryptosporidium parvum, Cyclospora, Microsporidia.*

DYSENTRY: It is characterized by diarrhea with increased blood and mucus, often associated with fever, abdominal pain and tenesmus. Causes are:

Bacterial: *Shigella* spp. *Campylobacter jejuni*, Enterohemorrhagic *E.coli*, Enterinvasine *E.coli*

Parasite: *Entamoeba histolytica, Balantidium coli.*

Q8. In an outbreak of suspected food poisoning, how is the food sample collected and transported to the laboratory? What are the common organisms causing?

Definition: Food poisoning refers to an illness acquired through consumption of food and drink contaminated either with microorganisms or their toxins.

During outbreaks vomitus, stool or suspected food materials are the ideal specimens. Food material should be homogenised or washed thoroughly in sterile diluent. e.g Ringer's solution.

Several non-bacterial agents that can cause food poisoning such as capsiacin , variety of toxins found in fish and shellfish, poisonous mushrooms and some chemical poisons.

Clinical manifestations and appearance of symptons within:

Within 1–6 hrs: *Stapylococcus aureus, Bacillus cereus, Clostridium botulinum.*

8–16 hrs: Clostridium perfringens, Bacillus cereus

>16 hrs: *Vibrio cholerae,* Enterotoxigenic *E.coli,* Enterohemorrhagic *E.coli, Salmonella* spp., *Campylobacter jejuni, Shigella* spp., *Vibrio parahemolyticus.*

Chapter 15 Serology

Q1. Enumerate the Antigen Antibody reactions used in serological diagnosis and give the principle of each.

Types of Antigen-antibody reactions

Conventional techniques:

- Precipitation reaction
- Agglutination reaction
- Complement fixation test
- Neutralisation test

Newer techniques (labelled assays):

- Enzyme linked immunosorbent assay (ELISA)
- Immunofluorescnce assay (IFA)
- Radioimmunoassay (RIA)
- Chemiluminescence—linked immunoassay (CLIA)
- Rapid test—Cassette ELISA, lateral flow test (immunochromatographic test), flow through assay.

Q2. What is precipitation and enumerate various precipitation reactions.

Definition:

When a soluble antigen reacts with its specific antibody in the presence electrolyte at optimal temperature and pH, it leads to formation of antigen-antibody complex in the form of:

*Insoluble precipitate band when gel containing medium is used or insoluble floccules or precipitate ring when liquid medium is used.

A. Precipitation in Liquid medium:

- Ring test: Ascoli's thermoprecipitin test , Streptococcal grouping by Lancefield's technique
- Slide test: Flocculation test–VDRL test for syphilis
- Tube test: Kahn's test for syphilis

B. Precipitation in gel (Immunodiffusion)

- Single diffusion in one dimension (Oudin Procedure)
- Double diffusion in one dimension (Oakley-Fulthorpe procedure)
- Single diffusion in two dimensions (Radial immunodiffusion)
- Double diffusion in two dimensions (Ouchterlony procedure)

C. Immunoelectrophoresis

D. Electroimmunodiffusion

- Countercurrent immunoelectrophoresis (CIEP)
- Rocket electrophoresis

Q.3 Define agglutination and enumerate various agglutination reactions.

Definition:

When a particulate or insoluble antigen is mixed with its specific antibody in the presence of electrolytes at a suitable temperature and pH, particles are clumped or agglutinated.

1. **Direct Agglutination test:**
   - *Slide agglutination test*—for blood grouping and cross matching
   - *Tube agglutination test*—Widal test for Enteric fever
   - *Hetrophile agglutination test:* Weil felix for Typhus fever, Paul Bunnel test for Infectious mononucleosis
   - *Microscopic agglutination*—for leptospirosis
   -
2. **Passive agglutination test (for antibody detection):**
   A precipitation reaction can be converted into agglutination test by attaching soluble antigens to the surface of carrier such as latex particles, bentonite and red blood cells.

   a. *Latex Agglutination test (LAT)* - for detection of ASO (antistreptolysin antibody), CRP, RA
   b. *Indirect Hemagglutination test*

3. **Reverse passive agglutination reaction:** When instead of antigen, antibody is absorbed on the carrier particles for detection of antigens.

   a. *Coagglutination test*: Staphylococcus aureus (protein A) acts as a carrier molecule. Specific antibody binds with Fc portion and Fab site remain free. Such sensitized cells are used for detection of antigen. Eg Salmonella typhi antigen in serum
   b. For detection of Hepatitis B surface antigen (HBsAg)

Q4. Describe the principle and applications of Coomb's test.

It is performed to diagnose Rh incompatability by detecting Rh antibody from mother's and baby's serum. It is used to test for autoimmune hemolytic anemia

Direct Coombs test (also known as the direct antiglobulin test or DAT) is used to detect if antibodies or complement system factors have bound to RBC surface antigens **in vivo**. A blood sample is taken and the RBCs are washed and then incubated with antihuman globulin. If this produces agglutination of RBCs, the direct Coombs test is **positive. Eg Erythroblastosis foetalis**

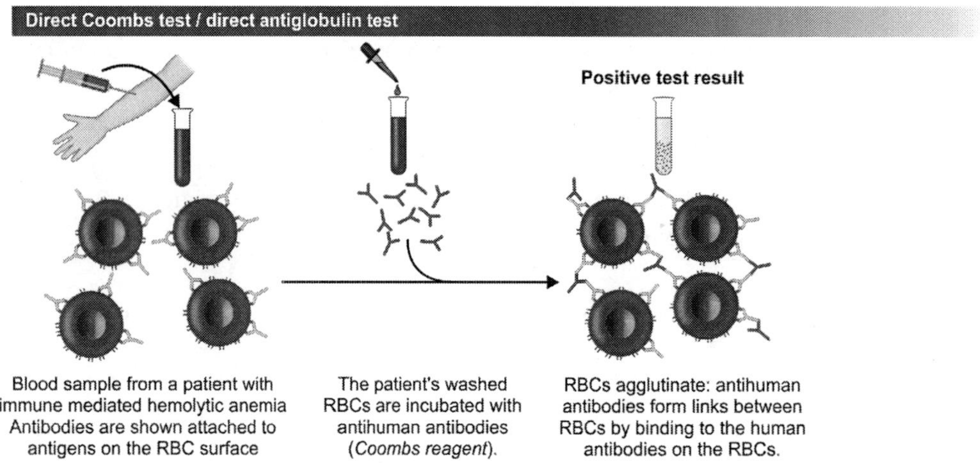

Indirect Coombs test (also known as the indirect antiglobulin test or IAT) is used to detect **in-vitro** antibody-antigen reactions. It is used to detect very low concentrations of antibodies present in a patient's plasma/serum prior to a blood transfusion. In antenatal care, this test is used to screen pregnant women for antibodies that may cause hemolytic disease of the newborn. The IAT can also be used for compatibility testing, antibody identification.

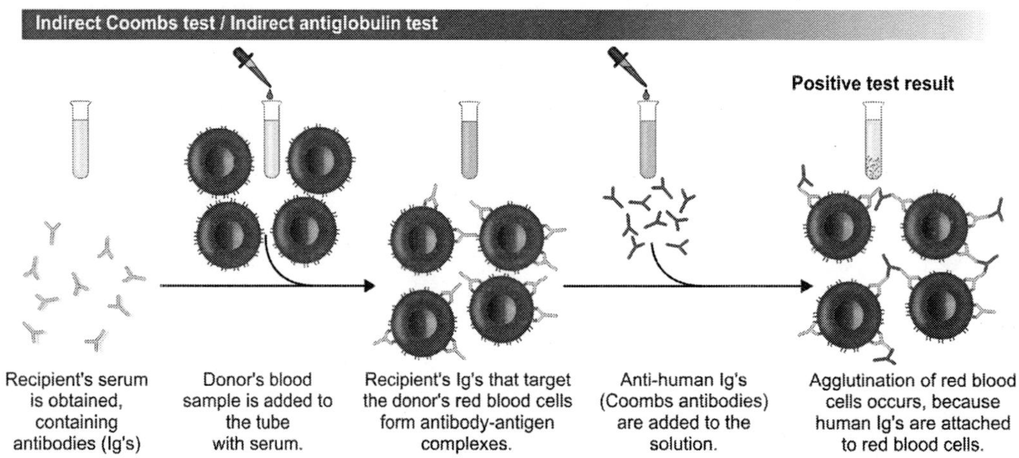

Q5. Tabulate the differences between precipitation and agglutination reactions.

Q.6 Write briefly about complement fixation test.

Principle: It is a two way step. When antigen and antibodies are mixed, complement is fixed to the antigen- antibody complex. It can be detected by adding amboreceptors (Sheep RBCs coated with anti sheep RBC antibody)

First Step

Antigen (soluble or particulate) + test serum + guinea pig complement are all added together.

If the test serum is positive for antibody, Ag-Ab complex is formed. Complement gets fixed to the complex, so there will be no free complements in the serum.

If the test serum is negative for antibody, there is no Ag-Ab complex. Complements are not fixed , hence remain free in the serum.

Second Step

A hemolysis indicator system is added . It consists of sheep RBCs coated with its antibodies called amboreceptors.

If the test serum is positive for antibody -------- no free complement in serum for binding to amboreceptors ---------- ***No hemolysis.***

If the test serum is negative for antibody ----------- free complement are attached to amboreceptors bound on sheep RBCs---------- ***Hemolysis.***

Q7. What is immunofluorescence and describe its techniuques. Mention their applications.

Principle: Fluorescence refers to absorbing high energy-shorter wavelength ultrviolet light rays by the fluorescent compounds and in turn emitting visible light rays with a low energy-longer wavelength. Commonly used fluorescent dyes are fluoroscien isothiocyanate, rhodamine.

Types of immunofluorescence tests are:

Direct immunofluorescence test: Specific antibodies tagged with fluorescent dye are used for detection of unknown antigen. If antigen is present, it reacts with labeled antibodies and fluorescence can be observed.

Indiract immunofluorescence assay: A known antigen is fixed on slide and unknown antibody in patient's serum attaches to the known antigen on the slide. For detection of antigen-antibody reaction, fluorescein tagged antibody to human globulin is added, thus which is observed under fluorescent microscope.

Applications

Detection of autoantibodies—(antinuclear antibody) in autoimmune diseases.
Detection of bacteria in blood, CSF, urine , faeces, tissue and other specimens.
Detection of microbial antigens—rabies antigen in corneal smear.
Detection of viral antigens in cell lines inoculated with the specimens.

Q8. Write briefly about radioimmunoassay (RIA). How is radioimmunoassay useful in diagnosis?

Radioimmunoassay (**RIA**) is an immunoassay that is based on competition for a fixed amounts of specific antibody between a known radiolabelled antigen and unknown unlabelled (test) antigen. After antigen- antibody reaction, antigen is separated into 'free' and 'bound' fractions and their radioactivity is measured.

It uses radiolabelled molecules in a stepwise formation of immune complexes. An RIA is a very sensitive in vitro assay technique used to measure concentrations of substances, usually measuring antigenconcentrations.

USES

- The test can be used to determine very small quantities (e.g. nanogram) of antigens and antibodies in the serum.
- The test is used for quantitation of hormones, drugs, HBsAg, and other viral antigens.
- Analyze nanomolar and picomolar concentrations of hormones in biological fluids.

Q9. Mention the principle of ELISA. Describe the different types of ELISA done. List out the various applications.

Principle: ELISA can provide a useful measurement of antigen or antibody concentration. There are two components:

Immunosorbent: An absorbing material (polyvinyl, polystyrene) is used that specifically absorbs the known antigen or antibody.

Enzyme: Is used to label one of the components of immunoassay.

Following antigen-antibody reaction, chromogenic substrate specific to enzyme (o-phenyldiaminefor peroxidase and p-nitrophenyl phosphate for alkaline phosphatase) is added. Reaction is detected by reading optical density.

(Ag+AB complex) - enzyme + substrate → activates the chromogen → color change → Detected by spectrophotometry

Types of ELISA

Direct ELISA: Used for detection of antigen.

Indirect ELISA: Used for detection of antibody/antigen.

Sandwich ELISA: Used for detection of antigen-Direct (single Ab) and Indirect (double Ab) Sandwich ELISA

Competitive ELSA: Used for detection of antigen/ antibody.

Cassette ELISA (Cylinder ELISA): Used for detection of antibody.

Applications

For antigen detection: Hepatitis B surface antigen, hepatitis B inner core antigen, NS1 dengue antigen

For antibody detection: Hepatitis B, C, HIV, Dengue, Epstein-Barr virus, Herpes simplex virus, Toxoplasmosis, Leishmaniasis.

SEROLOGY PRACTICAL EXCERCISE

Practical 1

Slide flocculation test: VDRL test

Practical 2

Slide agglutination test: Slide Widal test
Observe and interpret the given serological test.

Practical 3

IMMUNOASSAY : Cassette ELISA
Observe and interpret the given serological test

DELAYED HYPERSENSITIVITY TESTS FOR CELL MEDIATED IMMUNITY

Observe and interpret the skin tests in the given pictures.

Practical 1: Mantoux test.

Q1. Describe the process of phagocytosis and mention the various cells involved.

Q2. What is opsonisation?

Chapter **16**

Stool Examination

Aim: To do a microscopic examination of the given sample of stool and report.

Requirement: Normal saline, Lugol's iodine, Glass slides, Cover slips, Compound microscope, stool suspension. Composition of Lugol's Iodine:

Iodine crystals	-	1 g
Potassium iodine	-	2 g
Distilled water	-	100 mL

Procedure:

1. A drop of normal saline is placed on the centre of a clean slide.
2. About 2 mg of the given sample of stool is emulsified in the saline.
3. A cover slip is then placed on the emulsion avoiding air bubbles.
4. After reducing the light by lowering the condenser and using the concave mirror, the preparations first screened under low power.
5. When a cyst or an ovum is seen the details are observed by focussing under high power.
6. If cysts are seen, another preparation is made by emulsifying about 3 mg. of stool sample in Lugol's iodine. This helps to stain the nuclei.

Advantages of Iodine

- Lugol's iodine stain is intended to be used with wet mount preparations and concentration techniques for the detection of intestinal protozoa.
- Lugol's iodine is a rapid, non-specific contrast dye that is added to direct wet mounts of fecal material to aid in differentiating parasitic cysts from host white blood cells.
- Iodine stains protozoan nuclei and intracytoplasmic organelles brown making them easier to identify. It tends to paralyze the motility of parasitic organisms and may obscure some parasitic structures.

Chapter 17

Morphology of Various Parasites

1. Cyst of *Entamoeba histolytica*

- Quadrinucleate cyst, measures 18–40 μm in size
- Clear ectoplasm with granular endoplasm with erythrocytes and tissue debris found in vacuole
- It has a nucleus with central karyosome
- Trophozoite motile by pseudopodia.

2. Cyst of *Giardia lamblia*.

- Lives in duodenum and upper jejunum
- Oval ellipsoidal in shape with thick cyst wall
- Bilaterally symmetrical with two axostyles placed diagonally

Two pair of nuclei are also present

- Demonstration by Enterotest.

3. *Taenia saginata*

- Large, 5–10 mts in length
- Scolex is rhomboidal
- 2 mm in diameter
- Four suckers are present, pigmented
- Lacks rostellum and hooklets
- Bile stained ova seen

4. *Taenia solium*

- Small, 2-3 mts in length, globular
- Possess Rostellum and hooklets
- Suckers are not pigmented
- Bile stained ova.

5. Ovum of *Hymenolepis nana*

- Oval 30–45 μm in size
- Non bile stained
- Outer membrane is thin colourless, inner membrane (embryophore) encloses oncosphere
- 3 pairs of hooklets.

6. Fertilised egg of *Ascaris lumbricoides*

- Round to oval in shape, 60–75 μm in size
- Bile stained
- Surrounded by thick, transparent shell, consisting of vitelline membrane
- Outermost layer is coarsely, regular, albuminoid.

7. **Unfertilised egg of *Ascaris lumbricoides***

- Narrower and longer, 90 × 55 μm in size
- Bile stained
- Egg contains small atrophied ovum with thin shell within an irregular coating of albumin
- Heaviest of helminthic egg, do not float in saturated solution of common salt.

8. **Egg of *Ancylostoma duodenale***

- Oval and elliptical , 60 μm × 40 μm in size
- Non bile stained
- Possess a segmented ovum with four blastomeres
- Clear space between the segmented ovum and egg shell.

9. **Egg of *Enterobius vermicularis***

- Non bile stained
- Embryonated egg is the infective stage
- Egg shell is thin, hyaline, transparent, encloses larva.

10. Egg of *Trichuris trichiura*

- Eggs are barrel shaped with mucous plug at each other
- It is bile stained
- 50–54 μm in size
- Float in staurated solution of common salt.

11. Trypanosomes:

- Morphological forms—trypomastigote and amastigote
- Trypomastigote is infective form found in peripheral blood, C shaped 20 μm in size
- Kinetoplast is situated in the posterior end
- Stained by Giemsa and Wright stains.

12. *Leishmania donovani*:

- Morphological forms—LD bodies and promastigotes
- Promastigote—cells are elongated, posterior end is pointed
- Long flagellum projects from posterior end
- Amastigote form—resides in Reticuloendothelial system, is oval body measuring 2–4 μm in size, can be stained by
- Wright and Giemsa stain.

13. *Plasmodium vivax*:

- Staining with Giemsa/Romanowsky stain
- Cytoplasm shows signet ring appearance
- RBCS are enlarged, with portion of cytoplasm not occupied by parasite shows dotted or stippled appearance called Schuffner's dots—numerous fine golden brown in color.

14. *Plasmodium falciparum*:

- RBCs are normal in size
- Crescent shaped (banana shaped), long and slender gametocyte is seen
- Schizoint stage is absent
- Ring stage—small, delicate with 2 chromatin dots, one or more rings in one RBC.

15. Microfilariae (*Wuchereria bancrofti*)

- Transparent and colorless with blunt head and pointed tail
- Measures 250–300 μm in size, covered with hyaline sheath
- Somatic cells or nuclei appear as granules in the central axis of microfilaria
- Tail tip is free of nuclei.

Q1. Define zoonoses? Give Examples.

Definition:

Parasitic:

Bacterial:

Viral:

Fungal:

Q2. Enumerate intestinal protozoa.

Q3. How will you differentiate between the cysts of *E. histolytica* and *E. coli*?

Q4. Mention the extraintestinal lesions in amoebiasis.

Q5. What is P.A.M. (Primary Amoebic Meningoencephalitis)?

Q6. Enumerate the parasites affecting the liver.

Q7. List out the parasites affecting the central nervous system.

Q8. Enumerate the parasites affecting the lungs.

Q9. Name the various parasites affecting the genitourinary tract.

Q10. Name the parasites affecting the eyes.

Q11. Enumerate the parasites causing opportunistic infections.

Q12. Name the various parasites transmitted by penetration of the skin.

Q13. What are the parasites transmissible by blood transfusion?

Q14. Name the parasites that are sexually transmitted.

Q15. Name the parasites transmitted by vectors.

Q16. Name the parasites found in the peripheral blood smear.

Q17. Mention the infective forms of the following Protozoans.

Protozoan	*Infective forms*
Entamoeba histolytica	Tetranucleate cyst
Naegleria fowleri	Trophozoite
Acanthamoeba nigricans	Trophozoite and cyst
Giardia lamblia	Cyst
Trichomonas vaginalis	Trophozoite
Leishmania	Promastigote
Balantidium coli	Cyst
Plasmodium	Sporozoite
Toxoplasma gondii	Oocyst
Cryptosporidium	Oocyst and Tissue cyst

Q18. Mention the infective forms of the following Helminths.

Helminth	*Infective form*
Taenia	Cysticercous bovis (T. saginata) and Cysticercus cellulosae(T.solium)
Diphyllobothrium latum	Plerocercoid larvae
Echinococcus granulosus	Egg
Hymenolepis nana	Egg
Fasciola	Metacercaria larva
Paragonimus westermani	Metacercaria larva
Schistosoma	Cercaria larva
Ascaris lumbricoides	Egg
Ancylostoma duodenale	Filariform larva
Trichinella spiralis	Encysted larva
Strongyloides stercoralis	Filariform larva
Trichuris trichiura	Egg
Enterobius vermicularis	Egg
Filarial worms	3rd stage larva
Drancunculus medinensis	3rd stage larva

Q19. Define:

a. Viviparous parasites. Give examples.

b. Ovo-viviparous parasite. Give example.

c. **Oviparous parasites. Give examples.**

Q20. Name some bile stained Ova.

Q21. Name some non bile stained Ova.

Q22. Describe the concentration techniques used for stool examination.

Chapter **18**

Morphology of Fungi

Aim: To make a Lactophenol cotton blue preparation of the given fungal culture and report.

Requirements: Lactophenol cotton blue (LCB) solution.

Composition of Lactophenol cotton Blue:

- **Phenol crystals** – 20 g
- **Lactic acid** – 20 mL
- **Glycerol** – 40 mL
- **Distilled Water** – 20 mL
- **Cotton Blue** – 0.075 g

The phenol crystals are dissolved in the liquid by gently warming. Add dye to it.

Procedure:

1. A drop of Lactophenol cotton blue is placed on the center of a clean slide.
2. Using a sterile needle, a small portion of the pure fungal colony in the given culture is transferred to the drop of LCB slide.
3. It is then teased apart with dissecting needles.
4. A cover slip is carefully placed on the preparation avoiding air bubbles.
5. After reducing the light, by lowering the condenser and using the concave mirror, the preparation is first screened under low power to visualise the hyphae and the conidia.
6. It is then visualized under high power in order to identify the fungus.

KOH mount:

Potassium hydroxide (KOH) mount is a very useful test for the laboratory diagnosis of fungal infection of tissues especially skin, hair and nails. KOH separates the fungal elements from intact cells as it digests the protein debris and dissolves cement substances that holds the keratinized cells together and makes it easy to visualize under the microscope.

Requirements:

1. 10% KOH
2. Coverslip
3. Glass slide
4. Needle
5. Bunsen flame
6. Specimen

KOH Procedure

- Place the specimens like epidermal scales, nail, hair, skin scrapping or tissue on a clean glass slide.
- Pour a drop of 10% KOH on the specimen and place a converslip over it.
- Heat the slide gently over flame.
- Leave the slide for 5–10 minutes.
- Examine the slide under microscope.

Enumerate various fungi based on their morphology and draw suitable diagrams

1. ***Cryptococcus neoformans:***

- Capsulated yeast cell
- Demonstration of capsule by—negative staining by India ink
- Causes opportunistic infection Cryptococcosis
- CSF sample is taken

2. ***Candida albicans:***

- Ovoid or spherical budding yeast cells are seen on Gram staining
- Pseudohyphae—tube like elongations seen in tissue for invasion.
- Can cause opportunistic infections
- Germ tube test or Reynolds Braude phenomenon is seen

3. ***Trichophyton:***

- Segmented hyphae with conidia are seen on lactophenol cotton blue (LPCB) stain
- Microconidia—abundant, arranged along hyphae
- Macroconidia—scanty with blunt edges
- Infects skin, hair and nail

4. *Microsporum:*

- Segmented hyphae
- Microconidia are few and plenty of macroconidia are present
- Macroconidia—large, multicellular, spindle shaped
- Infects skin and hair

5. *Epidermophyton:*

- Microconidia are absent
- Macrocnidia are abundant—multicellular, pear shaped
- Infects skin and nails

6. *Madurella mycetomatis:*

- Pus from sinuses containing granules or grains is processed
- Granules—microcolonies of fungus
- LCB mount of crushed granules

7. **Rhinosporidium:**

- Large number of fungal spherules are seen
- Each spherule matures into a sporangium 350 μm in size
- Thousands of endospores(6–9 μm) in each sporangium
- *Rhinosporidium seeberi*—mainly seen as nasal mass

8. ***Aspergilus niger:***

- Grossly, colonies are black are in color
- Septate hyphae with condiophores are seen
- Vesicle is globular with uniseriate/biseriate sterigmata

9. ***Aspergillus fumigatus:***

- Grossly colonies are dark green in color
- Vesicle is conical in shape with uniseriate sterigmata
- Septate hyphae with condiophores are seen

10. *Penicillium:*

- Grossly colonies are blue-green in color with white border and a powdery surface
- Septate hyphae with branched conidiophores, with two rows of sterigmata bearing chain of spores—brush or broom appearance

11. *Mucor:*

- Broad aseptate hypahe are seen
- Sporangiophores are seen with sporangia and spores
- Rhizoids are absent

12. *Rhizopus:*

- Broad aseptate hyphae are seen
- Rhizoids are present

Q1. What are dermatophytes and classify them?

Q2. Name the fungi responsible for Subcutaneous mycotic infections.

Q3. What are the various causative agents of Mycetoma? Mention the differences between bacterial and fungal (Eumycotic) Mycetomas.

Q4 What are dimorphic fungi? Give examples.

Q5. Mention the various specimens, possible fungal pathogens and their methods of demonstration in the following clinical conditions:

Disease	*Specimen*	*Possible fungal pathogens*	*Method of demonstration*
Dermatophytosis	**Skin, hair and nail**		
Meningitis	**CSF**		
Keratomycosis	**Corneal scrappings**		
Otomycosis	**Ear swab**		
Nasal polyps	**Nasal mucosa scrappings**		
Resp tract Infection	**Sputum**		
Vaginitis	**Vaginal swab**		
Mycetoma	**Pus with granules**		
Systemic mycoses	**Sputum, bone marrow biopsy, blood**		

Q6. Mention some media used for the isolation of fungi in the laboratory.

Q7. What is the composition of Sabouraud's Dextrose Agar (SDA)?

Q8. What are the antimicrobial agents added to SDA.

a. While isolating dermatophytes?

b. While isolating fungi causing systemic infections?

Q9. What is 'ID' reaction?

Q10. What are Mycotoxins? Give any two examples

Q11. What are opportunistic fungal infections? Mention the various conditions that predispose to such infections.

Q12. What are dematiaceous fungi? Give examples.

Chapter 19 Morphology of Viruses

A. Describe with suitable diagrams the DNA viruses represented by the given models:

1. Pox virus:

- Brick-shaped, largest DNA virus
- Grows in chorioallantoic membrane (CAM)
- Small pox virus (Variola virus),Vaccinia virus
- Produce pocks on CAM in 48–72 hrs

2. Herpes virus:

- Icosahedral symmetry, 150–200 nm in diameter
- Lipid envelope with peplomers
- Tegument present between capsid and peplomers
- ***Tzanck cells*** (multinucleated giant cells with faceted nuclei and homogenously stained ground glass chromatic) in HSV-2

3. Adenovirus:

- Non-enveloped, 70–90 nm in diameter
- Icosahedral in symmetry with 252 capsomers
- Fiber protein projecting from each vertex—space vehicle appearance
- Causes respiratory tract infections

4. Hepadnavirus:

- Enveloped virus with 42 nm in diameter
- Exists in three morphological forms—spherical, tubular and complete dane particle
- Envelope containing HbsAg surrounds partially double stranded DNA
- DNA dependent DNA polymerase enzyme is present

B. Describe with suitable diagrams the RNA viruses represented by the given models:

1. Picornavirus:

- Non-enveloped virus, spherical shaped
- Icosahedral capsid, 60 capsomere present
- Each capsid has 4 viral proteins, possess ssRNA
- Contains Enterovirus (Poliovirus) and Rhinovirus

2. Orthomyxovirus:

- Enveloped , spherical virus
- Helical symmetry
- ssRNA segmented in 8 pieces
- Nucleoprotein is major capsid protein, associated with RNA to form ribonucleoprotein

3. Rhabdovirus:

- Bullet shaped virus with one end rounded and other end flat (75 nm × 180 nm)
- Lipoprotein envelope with hemagglutinin spikes
- M layer present lines the envelope
- Nucleocapsid has helical symmetry, has ss negative sense RNA

4. Retrovirus:

- Enveloped virus (HIV)
- Possess enzyme reverse transcriptase which directs synthesis of DNA from viral RNA after infecting host cell
- 80–110 nm in diameter
- Icosahedral capsid made up of core protein

Chapter 20 Cultivation and Identification of Viruses

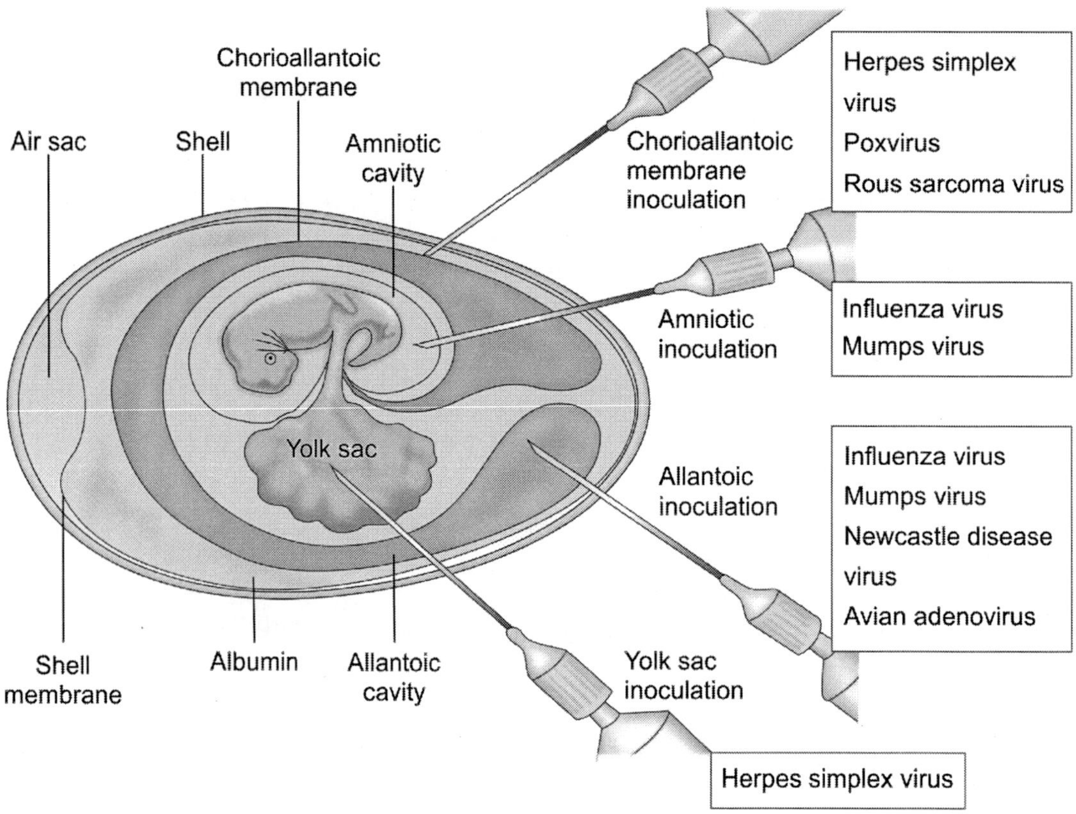

Growth of viruses in embryonated egg:
An embryonated chicken egg showing the different compartments in which viruses may grow. The different routes by which viruses are inoculated into eggs are indicated.

I. SPECIMENS OBTAINED FOR THE ISOLATION OF VIRUSES IN THE LABORATORY

Clinical manifestations	*Viruses suspected*	*Specimen collected*
Upper Respiratory Tract Infections	**Influenza , Parainfluenza, RSV, Adenovirus, Enterovirus**	
Lower Respiratory Tract Infections	**Respiratory syncytial virus, Parainfluenza**	
CNS Infections	**Arbovirus, Enterovirus, Rabies virus, Herpesvirus, Mumps**	
Conjunctivitis	**Herpes simplex virus, Herpes zoster virus, Adenovirus, Enterovirus**	
Serum hepatitis	**Hepatitis B, C, D**	
AIDS	**Human immunodeficiency virus**	
Infantile diarrhea	**Rotavirus, Calicivirus, Norwalkvrus, Astrovirus**	
Parotitis	**Mumps virus**	
Cutaneous and mucous membrane disease	**Varicella zoster virus, Measles and Cowpox**	

Q1. What is cytopathogenic effect (CPE)?

Q2. Define inclusion bodies. Give examples.

Cytoplasmic :

Nuclear :

Q3. List out the viruses which affect the respiratory system.

Upper respiratory tract:

Lower respiratory tract:

Q4. Enumerate the viruses causing gastroenteritis.

Q5. Mention the viruses affecting the central nervous system.

Q6. Mention the viral infections transmitted by sexual contact.

Q7. Mention the viral diseases that are congenitally transmitted.

Q8. What are teratogenic viruses? Give examples.

Q9. Name some oncogenic viruses.

Q10. What are arboviruses? Enumerate the arboviruses prevalent in India.

Q11. Mention some human slow viral infections.

Chapter 21

Applied Exercise

CASE STUDY-1

A 5-year-old child with fever and soreness of throat also develops difficulty in breathing. A throat swab collected is subjected to culture and a direct smear made is stained with Albert's technique. An vitro toxigenicity test also done.

A. Suggestive Organism:

Corynebacterium diphtheriae, which on Albert's staining shows Chinese letter pattern/Cuneiform arrangement (V or L shaped) with metachromatic granules and greenish cytoplasm.

B. Culture Media Used:

Loeffler's Serum slope, Tinsdale medium and Potassium tellurite agar.

C. Clinical Manifestation of Diphtheria:

- Respiratory Diphtheria
- Cutaneous Diphtheria
- Systemic Complications

D. Various tests for Diphtheria toxin demonstration:

- In vivo tests: Subcutaneous and intracutaneous tests
- In vitro tests: Elek's gel precipitation test, Detection of TOX gene by PCR

E. Prophylaxis:

- DPT vaccine at 6,10,14 weeks given IM
- Passive immunization—500 to1000 units of anti-diphtheritic serum (ADS)

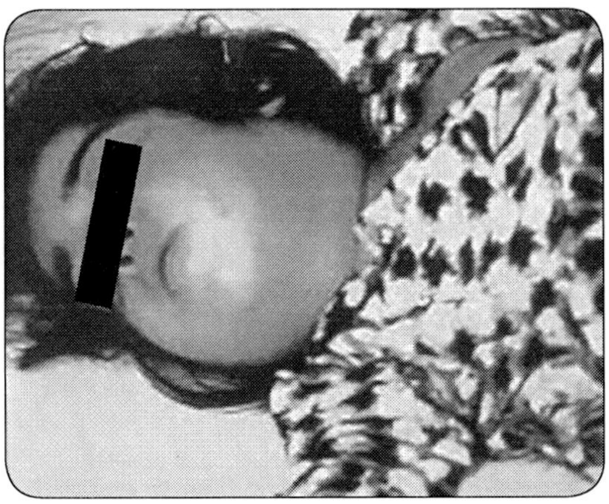

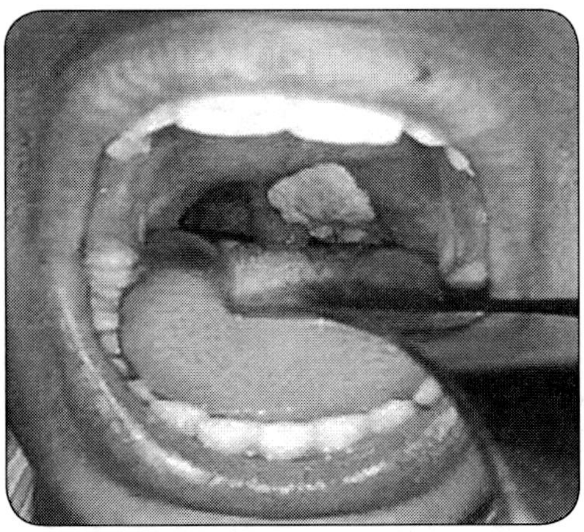

CASE STUDY-2

A 30-year-old female gives a history of low grade fever, cough with expectoration and mild pain in the chest since 1 year. A sputum specimen is collected for direct smear examination and for concentration and culture.

Causative organism: *Mycobacterium tuberculosis.*

Morphology:

Red colored, straight, slightly curved rod shaped bacilli of 3 × 0.3 microns.

Culture medium:

- Egg based (Lowenstein Jensen, Dorset, Petragnini)
- Agar based (Middlebrook 7H10 and 7H11)
- Liquid based (Middlebrook 7H12, Dubos, Proskauer and beck, Sulas and Sauton)
- Blood based (Tarshis)
- Potato based agar (Pawlowsky)

Automated Methods: Middle brook 7H10/7H11 available but mostly used in Automated systems–

- BACTEC 460
- SEPTI CHECK
- BACTEC MGIT 960
- BacT/Alert 3D

Clinical features: Cough with expectoration, hemoptysis, dyspnea, fever with chills and rigor, weight loss and night sweats.

Prophylaxis

BCG is given intradermal on anterior aspect of arm.

Diagnostic algorithm for pulmonary TB : New guideline

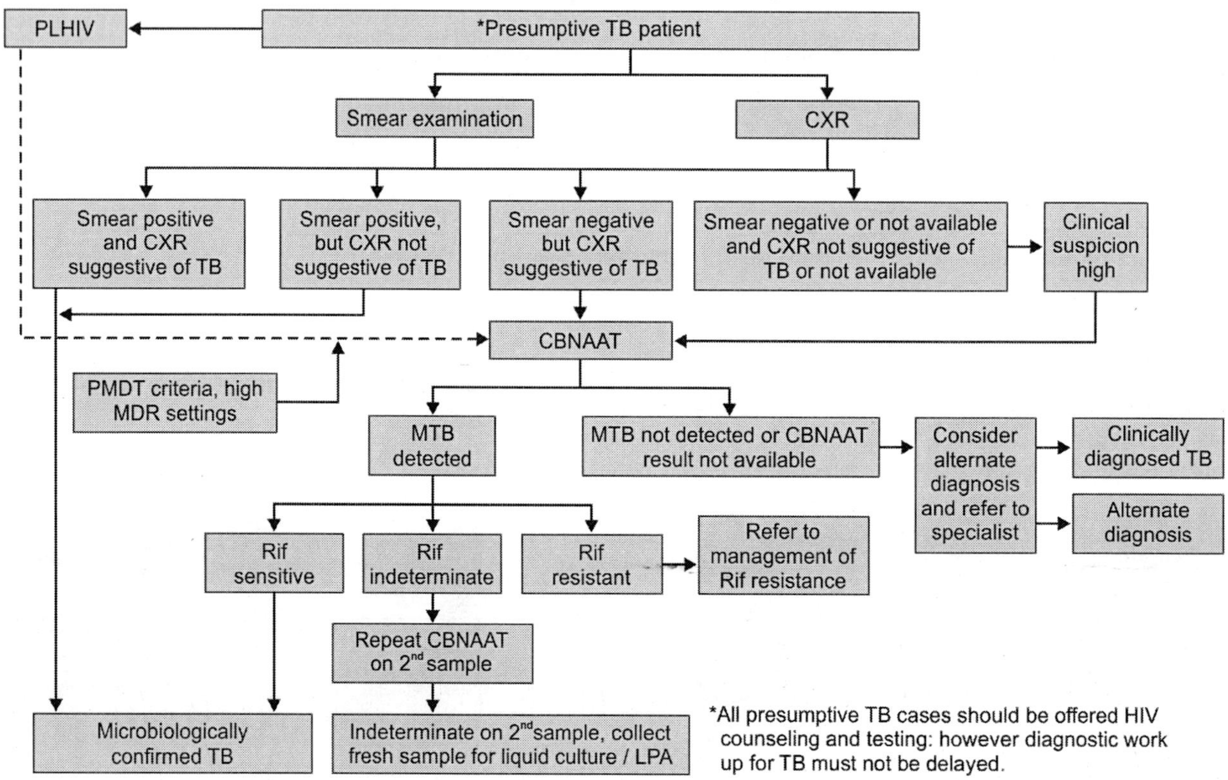

*All presumptive TB cases should be offered HIV counseling and testing: however diagnostic work up for TB must not be delayed.

CASE STUDY-3

A 30-year-old female comes to the outpatient department complaining of burning micturition and fever with chills and rigor. A midstream urine sample collected aseptically is subjected to culture and biochemical reactions were illustrated.

Causative organism: *Escherichia coli* causing UTI

Other causative organism are:

- *Gram positive: Staphylococcus aureus, S. saprophyticus, S. epidermidis* and *Enterococcus*
- *Gram negative: Klebsiella, Proteus, Pseudomonas* and *Citrobacter*
- *Fungus: Candida albicans* in diabetes and immunocompromised patients

Culture media: Blood agar, MacConkey's agar, CLED agar

Biochemical reactions of *E.coli*:

Catalase (+), Oxidase (-), Indole (+), Methyl red (+), Voges Prosker (-), Citrate (-), Urease (-)

TSI—ferments glucose, lactose and sucrose with acid gas production (A/A with or without gas)

Also ferments Maltose, Mannitol

Significant Bacteriuria: (Kass criteria)

Presence of bacteria more than 10^5CFU/mL in a mid stream urine sample by standard loop technique on MacConkey's agar. It indicates active/acute infection.

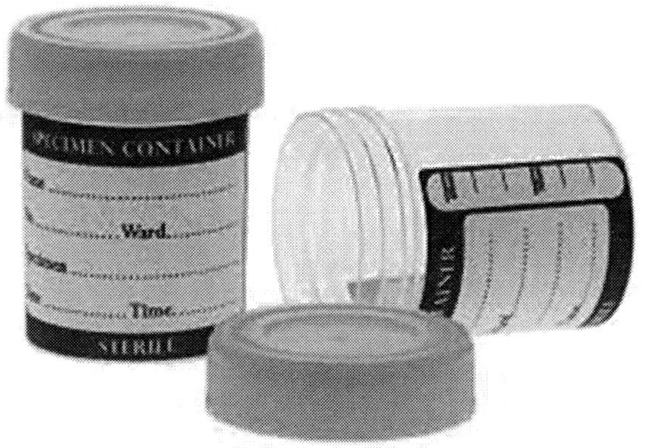

CASE-4

A 25-year-old female with a history of having delivered at home on the previous day, is brought to Emergency room. On examination, she has a temperature of 104°F, a rapid pulse and hypotension. Blood is collected for culture and the patient is started on antibiotic therapy. The broth is inoculated on solid media. Biochemical reactions are also put up.

Condition is: Gram negative septicemia

Causative organism are:

- *Gram positive: Staphylococcus aureus, Streptococcus pyogenes, Listeria monocytogenes*
- *Gram negative: Neisseria meningitidis, Salmonella typhi, Salmonella paratyphi* A, B, *Brucella, E.coli, Klebsiella, Proteus, Enterobacter.*

Pathogenesis of Endotoxic shock:

Lipopolysaccharide in cell wall of the gram negative bacteria produces the shock. Inactivates monocytes, macrophages which produce TNF which induces IL-1, TNF- α. IL-1 acts on endothelial cells to produce further cytokines IL-6 and which enhances inflammatory reactions.

Endotoxic shock is characterized by fever, leucopenia, thrombocytopenia, hypotension, circulatory shock leading to death.

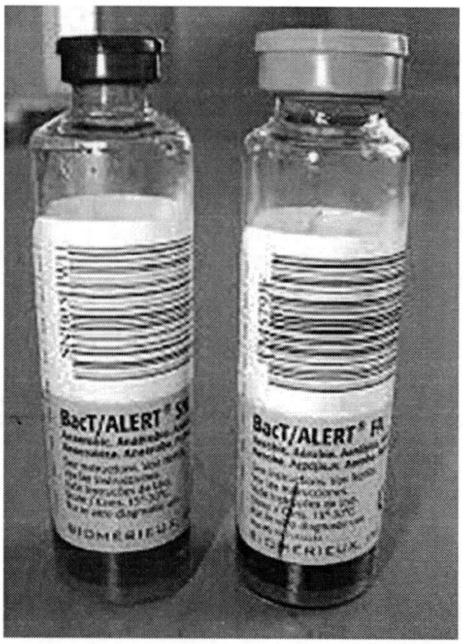

CASE-5

A 50-year-old male admitted to Medicine ward with history of fever since 8 days. On admission, blood culture was sent and serological testing was also performed.

Diagnosis and Causative organism: Enteric fever by *Salmonella typhi.*

Sample collection: Blood sample in blood culture bottle is collected before administering antibiotics. Using sterile syringe, 5-10 mL blood is collected for adults.

Media used for subculturing blood:

- Nutrient agar: Translucent colonies
- Nutrient agar: Pale colonies
- Blood agar: Grey coloured colonies
- Mac Conkey agar: Non-lactose fermenting colonies
- Wilson and Blair media: Jet black colnies with metallic sheen

Biochemical reactions: Catalase (+), Oxidase (-), Indole (-), Methyl red (+), Voges Prosker (-), Citrate (+), TSI - K/A with H_2S production at the junction of slant and butt. Glucose, Maltose and Mannitol is fermented

Serological testing: Widal test is done by second week of fever.

Other specimens collected are: Stool, urine, pus from roseolar rash, bone marrow, duodenal aspirates

Kauffman and White Scheme of Classification

- Antigenic notation: consists of 3 parts

a. O antigen: In arabic numerals

b. Phase-1 H antigen: a to z and then z1 to z83

c. Phase-2 H antigen: arabic numerals 1-12

O-ag	Serogroup	Serotype	O anigens	H antigen	
				Phase-1	Phase–2
2	A	S. Paratyphi A	1, 2, 12	a	(1, 5)
4	B	S. Paratyphi B	1, 4, (5), 12	b	1, 2
7	C1	S. Paratyphi C	6, 7(vi)	c	1, 5
9	D	S. Typhi	9, 12(vi)	d	–

CASE-6

A serological test is put up for a patient suffering from of 10 days duration. Interpret.

Test done: Widal tube agglutination test

Timing of test is important, as antibodies begin to arise during end of first week. The titers increase during second, third and fourth week after which it gradually declines. The test may be negative in early part of first week.

Principle:

Patients' suffering from enteric fever would possess antibodies in their sera which can react and agglutinate serial doubling dilutions of killed, coloured Salmonella antigens in a tube agglutination test.

Requirements: Widal rack, round-bottomed Felix tubes, conical-bottomed Dreyer's tubes, water bath, doubly diluted patient serum in three-four rows, Killed coloured suspensions of *S.typhi* O antigen, *S.typhi* H antigen, *S.paratyphi* AH antigen and optionally *S.paratyphi* BH antigen.

Reading the results: The control tubes must be examined first, where they should give no agglutination.

- Agglutination of O antigen appears as a "matt" or "carpet" at the bottom. Agglutination of H antigens appears loose, wooly or cottony. The highest dilution of serum that produces a positive agglutination is taken as titer. The titers for all the antigens are noted.
- Baseline titer of the population must be known before attaching significance to the titers. The antibody levels of individuals in a population of a given area give the baseline titer.
- **A titer of 100 or more for O antigen is considered significant and a titer in excess of 200 for H antigens is considered significant.**
- Patients who have received vaccines against *Salmonella* **may give false positive reactions**. True untreated infection results in rise in titer whereas vaccinated individuals do not demonstrate any rise in titer.
- **Anamnestic response:** Those individuals, who had suffered from enteric fever in the past, sometimes develop anti-Salmonella antibodies during an unrelated or closely related infection. It can be differentiated from true infection by lack of any rise in titre on repetition after a week.

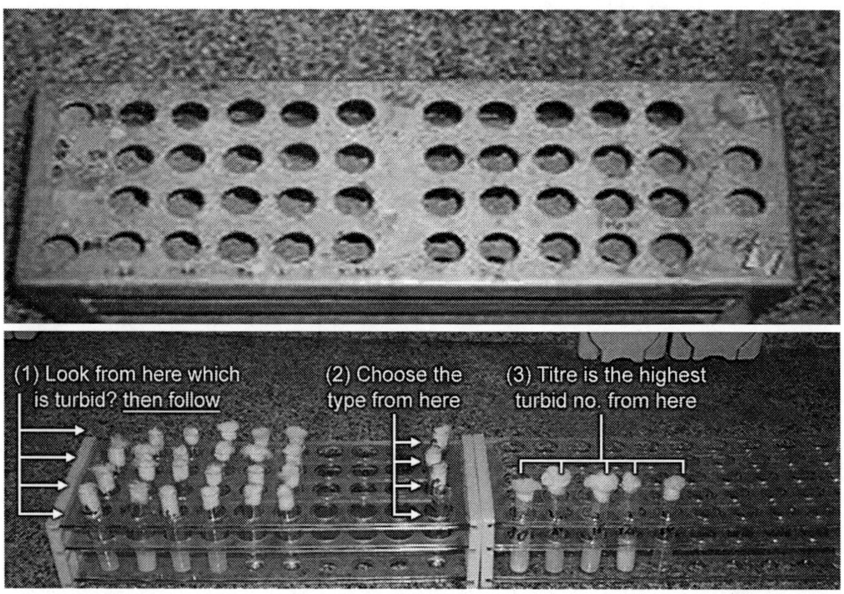

CASE-7

A 25-year-old male presents to the medical outpatient department with a history of jaundice of 1 month duration. Blood collected is subjected to electron microscopy and serological testings.

Causative organism: Hepatitis B

Particles seen on Electron Microscope are:

- Abundant spherical particles of 20 nm in diameter
- Tubular particles—200 nm in diameter
- Double shelled particle—Dane particle—42 nm in size, spherical.

Serological Testings done: Immunochromatographic tests, ELISA can be done.

- Anitgen markers: HBsAg, HBeAg, HBcAg
- Antibody marker: Anti-HBs, Anti- HBE and Anti- HBc
- Molecular markers: HBV DNA
- Non-specific markers: Elevated liver enzymes and serum bilirubin.

Prophylaxis:

- Recombinant subunit vaccine (3 doses-0,1 and 6 months)
- Hepatitis B Immunoglobulin (HBIG)—0.05-0.07 mL/kg body weight

Complications of serum hepatitis:

Hepatocellular carcinoma, Cirrhosis, Arthralgia, Urticaria, Polyarthritis, Glomerulonephritis

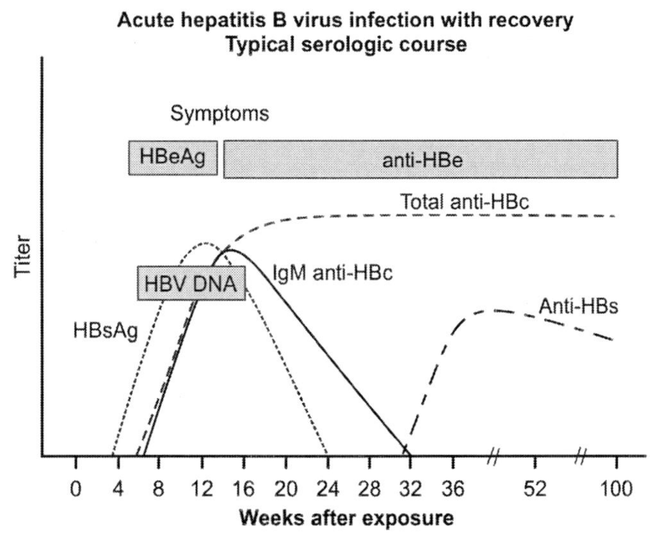

CASE-8

Blood donated by a 25-year-old male for a relative posted for surgery is found to be seropositive for HIV. He is referred to the laboratory for a confirmatory testing.

Characteristic feature of HIV:

- 80–110 nm in size, enveloped virus. Envelope is made up of:
  - Lipid part: Host cell membrane derived
  - Protein part: Glycoprotein 120 (gp-120) and Glycoprotein 41 (gp-41)
  - Nucleocapsid: Icosahedral in symmetry, made up of core protein, Inner core encloses two identical copies of ss positive linear RNA

Laboratory testing:

Specific tests for HIV infection

- Screening tests (ERS) (antibody detection): ELISA/Rapid test/Simple test
- Supplemental tests (antibody detection): Western blot, Immunofluorescence, Radioimmunoprecipitation assay

Confirmatory tests:

- p24 antigen detection
- Viral culture
- HIV RNA by Reverse transcriptase-PCR, Real-time PCR for estimating viral load
- Branched DNA assay
- Nucleic acid sequence based amplification (NASBA)
- HIV DNA testing for pediatric patients is confirmatory test.

Non-specific tests for HIV detection:

- Low CD4 T cell count
- Hypergammaglobulinemia
- Altered CD4:CD8 ratio.

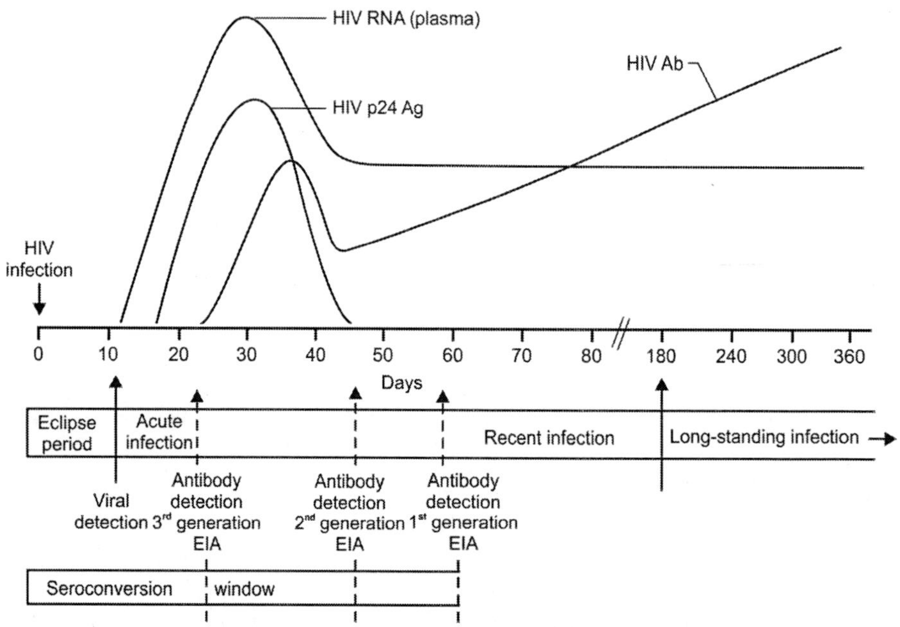

CASE-9

A 16-year-old male patient suffering from fever with rigors and loss of consciousness was brought to Medicine Emergency. A peripheral blood smear was made and other investigations were done. Thick and thin smears were made.

Causative organism: *Plasmodium falciparum*

Different stains used are: Giemsa, Leishman, Romanowsky, Wright's and Jaswant Singh Bhattacharya stain

- Thick smear: For Identification of malaria
- Thin smear: For species identification.
- Occurrence of multiple rings with accole formation—diagnostic of *P. falciparum*

Quantitative buffy coat: Acridine orange (AO) binds deoxyribonucleic acids and ribonucleic acids. The malaria parasite binds acridine orange in the nucleus and the cytoplasm and emits green and red fluorescence when excited at 480 nm allowing the detection and examination of parasite morphology by fluorescent microscopy.

Rapid diagnostic tests: RDTS for detection of antigen. Antigens targeted by RDTS are:

- Histidine rich protein-II (HRP-II)
- Parasite lactate dehydrogenase (pLDH)
- Aldolase

Complications: Anemia, Hemoglobinuria, Hemoglobinemia, Black water fever, Acute renal failure, Tropical splenomegaly, Cerebral malaria, Hypoglycemia

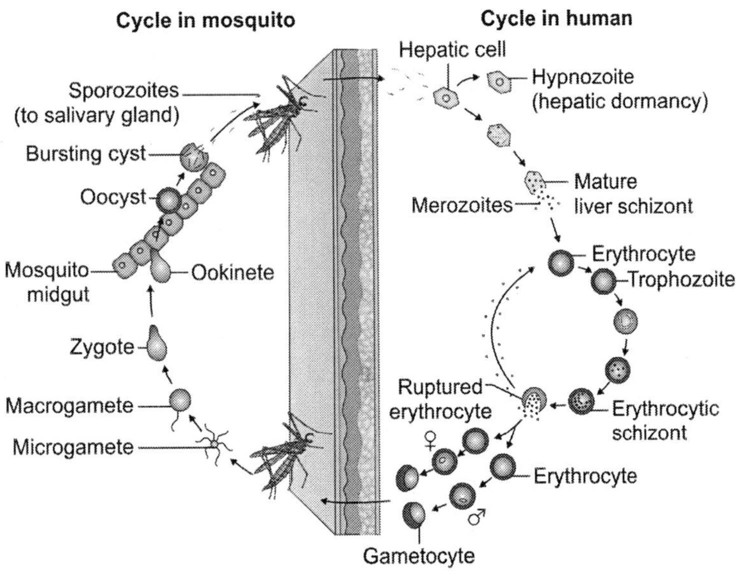

CASE-10

A 30-year-old female comes to the outpatient department complaining of curdy white discharge per vagina associated with intense pruritis. A high vaginal swab collected with aseptic precautions is subjected to culture and a smear made is stained by Gram's technique.

Causative organism: *Candida albicans*

Culture Media used: Sabouraud's dextrose agar. It can also grow on Blood agar.

Gram staining: Oval budding yeast cells are seen with pseudohyphae.

Confirmatory tests:

- *Germ tube test:* Pooled human sera when mixed with a colony of *C. albicans*, kept at 37°C for 2 hrs-- Tube like projections (Reynolds-Braude Phenomenon)
- Dalmau plate culture
- CHROM agar
- Sugar assimilation tests
- Immunodiagnosis: Cell wall Mannan antigen detection
- Molecular methods

Various lesions caused by *Candida albicans:*

- Mucosa candidiasis: Oral thrush, Vulvovaginitis, balanitis, Esophageal candidiasis, angular stomatitis
- Pulmonary Candidiasis
- Cutaneous Candidiasis: Paronychia, Intertrigo, Diaper candidiasis
- Invasive candidiasis: UTI, Septicemia, Keratitis, Keratoconjunctivitis, Nosocomial

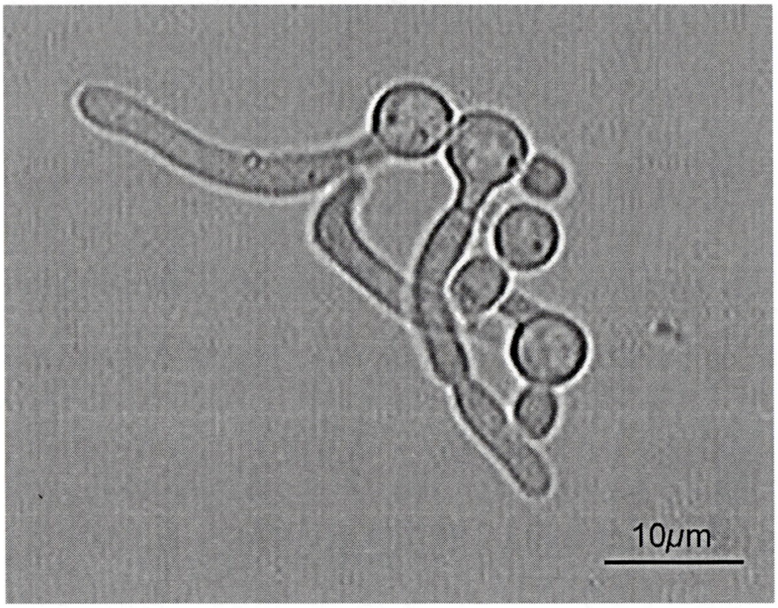

CASE-11

A 40-year-old male patient came with complaints of convulsions, headache and vomiting. CSF examination was performed and sample was subjected to culture and biochemical reactions.

Causative agent: *Cryptococcus neoformans*

Staining:

On Negative staining round: Modified India Ink capsule is demonstrated as refracted delineated clear space surrounding the round budding yeast cells are seen

On Gram staining: Round budding yeast cells are seen

Culture Media and biochemicals used:

Sabouraud dextrose agar without antibiotics, Niger seed agar, Bird seed agar

Urease is positive

Assimilation of inositol and nitrate

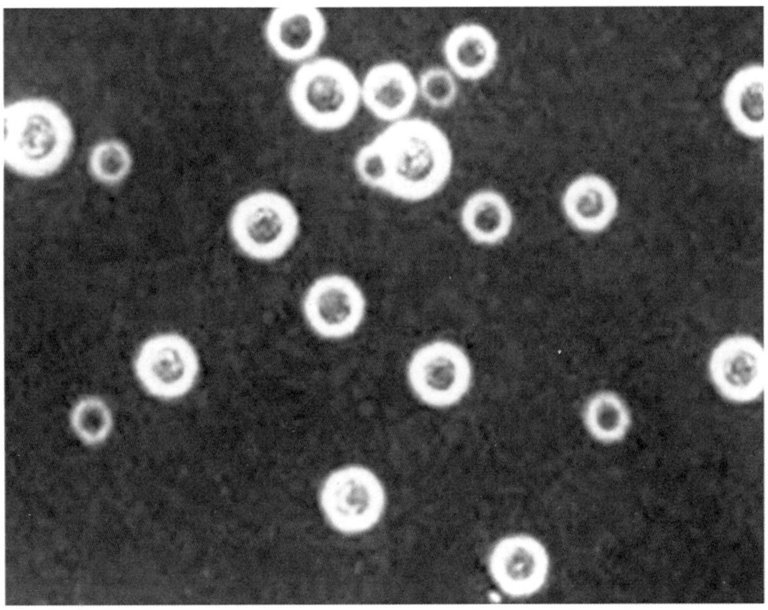

Chapter 22 Hospital Waste Management

Table 22.1: Biomedical waste management

Category	*Type of bag/container used*	*Type of waste*	*Treatment/Disposal options*
Yellow 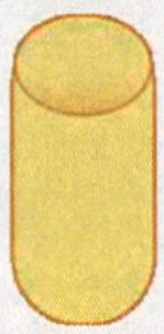	Non-chlorinated plastic bags Separate collection system leading to effluent treatment system	a. Human anatomical waste b. Animal anatomical waste c. Soiled waste d. Expired or discarded medicines e. Chemical waste f. Micro- Bio-T and other clinical lab waste g. Chemical liquid waste	Incineration or plasma Pyrolysis or deep burial
Red 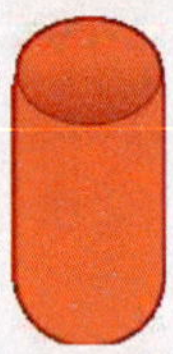	Non-chlorinated plastic bags or containers	i. Contaminated waste (recyclable) tubing, bottles, intravenous tubes and sets, catheters, urine bags, syringes (without needles) and gloves	Auto/Micro/Hydro and then sent for recycling not be sent to landfill
White 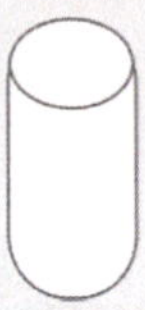	(Translucent) Puncture, leak, tamper-proof containers	Waste sharps including metals	Auto or dry heat sterillization followed by shredding or mutilation or encapsulation
Blue 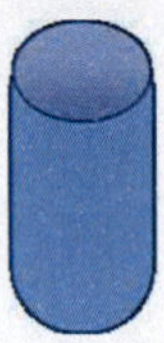	Cardboard boxes with blue colored marking	Glassware	Disinfection or auto/micro/hydro and then sent for recycling

Table 22.2: Color-coded bags for biomedical waste segregation as per 2016 rules

Category of bag	*Type of waste*	*Waste treatment*
Yellow 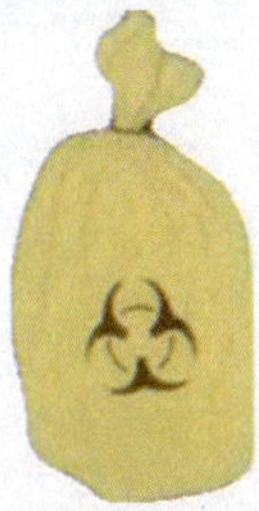	a. Human anatomical waste	Incineration or plasma pyrolysis or deep burial
	b. Animal anatomical waste	
	c. Soiled waste	Incineration or plasma pyrolysis or deep burial
	d. Expired or discarded medicines	Returned back to the manfacturer or supplier for incineration at temperature >12000°C
	e. Chemical waste	Incineration or plasma pyrolysis or deep burial or encapsulation
	f. Chemical liquid waste	Pretreatment and then disposal
	g. Discarded linen, mattresses, beddings contaminated with blood or body fluids	Nonchlorinated chemical disinfection followed by incineration or plasma pyrolysis
	h. Microbiology, biotechnology and other clinical laboratory waste	Pretreat to sterilize with nonchlorinated chemicals on-site as per NACO or WHO guidelines thereafter for incineration
Red 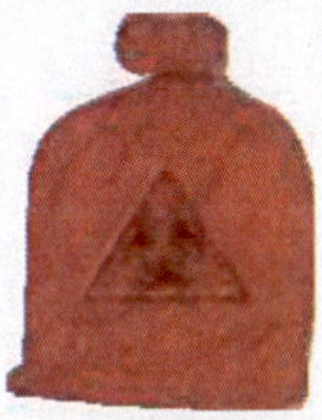	i. Contaminated waste (recyclable) like plastic bag, bottles, pipes or containers	Autoclaving or microwaving/hydroclaving followed by shredding of mutilation Treated waste to be sent to registered or autoclaved recyclers or for energy recoverry of plastics to diesel or fuel oil or for road-making
White translucent 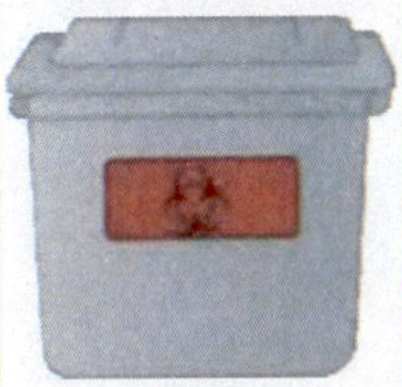	Waste sharps including metals: Needles, syringes with fixed needles, needles from needle tip cutter or burner, scalpels, blades	Autoclaving or dry-heat sterilization; followed by shredding or mutilation or encapsulation in metal container or cement concrete Sent for final disposal to iron foundries (having consent to operate from the state pollution control committees) Or sanitary landfill or designated concrete waste sharp pit
Blue cardboard box with blue label 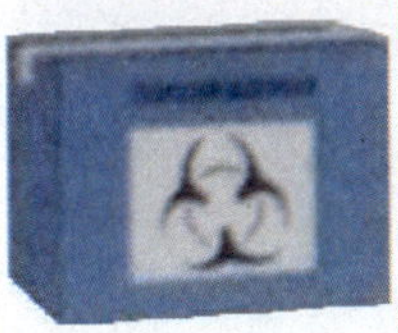	Glassware: Broken or discarded and contaminated glass including medicine vials and ampoules except those contaminated with cytotoxic wastes; metallic body implants	Disinfection (by soaking the washed glass waste after cleaning with deterged and sodium hypochlorite treatment) or through autoclaving or microwaving or hydroclaving; then sent for recycling

Chapter 23 Hand Hygiene

7 STEPS OF HAND WASHING

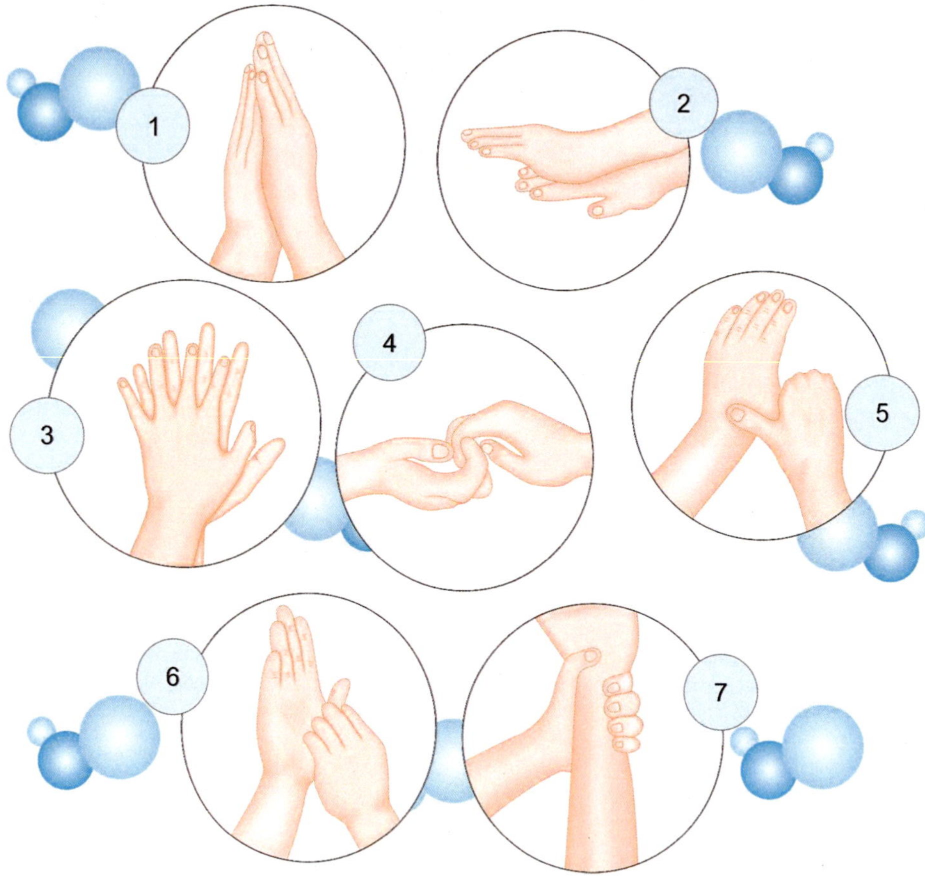

YOUR 5 MOMENTS

For **hand hygine**

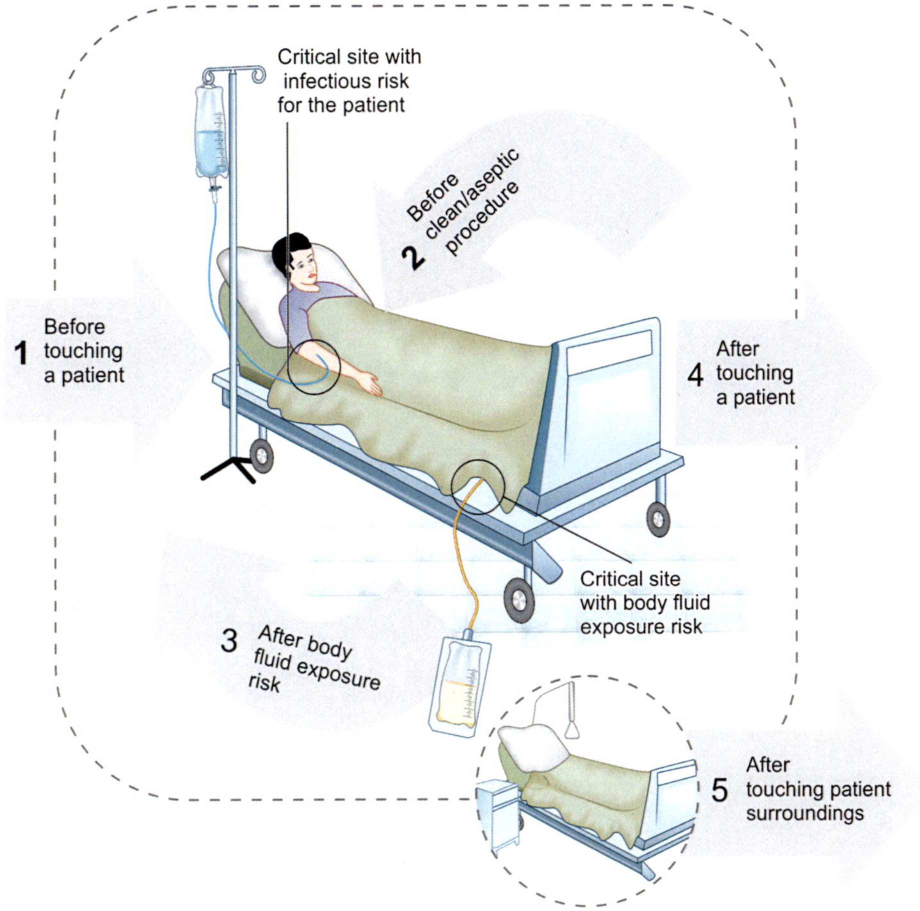